Doria Gani

Doria Gani is a Naked Yoga teacher and an ambassador for body positivity. She started practising yoga in 2010, as a form of rehabilitation after fighting cervical cancer. From that beginners' class, she found that the clear, mindful asana instructions improved her memory, spatial relations, focus, and sense of connectedness with her mind and body. On a greater scale, the daily practice showed her the value of acting deliberately. Yoga was the key to her recovery and transformation, and now she lives her life with a greater sense of purpose and intention.

Now qualified as a yoga teacher in Ashtanga Vinyasa, Rocket Yoga, Yin, Mandala, and principles of Ayurveda and Shamanism, Doria teaches Naked Yoga classes online as well as all around the world.

Doria has been featured on the BBC, East London Film Festival and in many press articles including in *Cosmopolitan, H&E Naturist, The Sun, Unreported London, The Londonist,* the *i* and *OM Yoga* Magazine.

www.doriayoga.com

Steve Robson

Steve is a successful entrepreneur who joined Doria Gani's Naked Yoga classes two years ago and found it helpful to reconnect with his body, improve his energy and enhance his spirituality.

www.brumbymediagroup.com

First published in the UK in 2021 by SUPERNOVA BOOKS
67 Grove Avenue, Twickenham, TW1 4HX

Supernova Books is an imprint of Aurora Metro Publications Ltd.
www.aurorametro.com @aurorametro FB/AuroraMetroBooks

Instagram @aurora_metro

The Naked Yoga Effect: From Cancer Survivor To Naked Yoga Teacher text copyright © 2021 Doria Gani & Steve Robson

Images: Lorenzo Lessi, Roberto Nencini, Ranger Ric, Maurizio Cecchini, Pink Agency, Alessandro Sigismondi, www.vallejoopenstudios.com

Sun Salutations graphic courtesy of Souvik Maity

Artwork R-evolution by Marco Cochrane www.marcocochranesculpture.net/r-evolution

Editor: Cheryl Robson

Printed in the UK by Short Run Press, Exeter, UK.

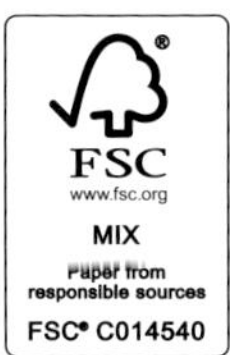

ISBNs:
978-1-913641-11-5 (print version)
978-1-913641-12-2 (ebook version)

The Naked Yoga Effect

From Cancer Survivor To Naked Yoga Teacher

by

Doria Gani

& Steve Robson

SUPERNOVA BOOKS

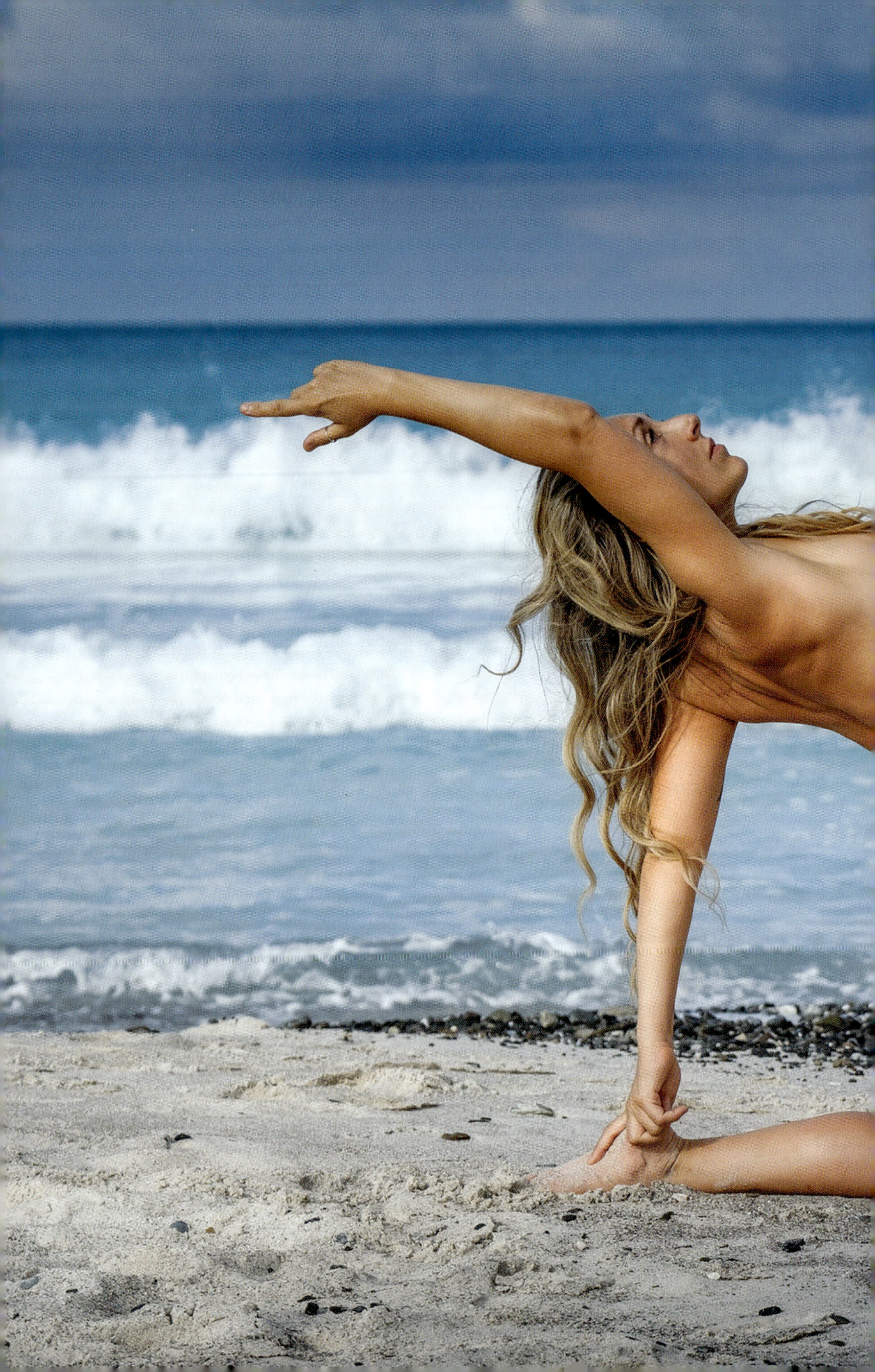

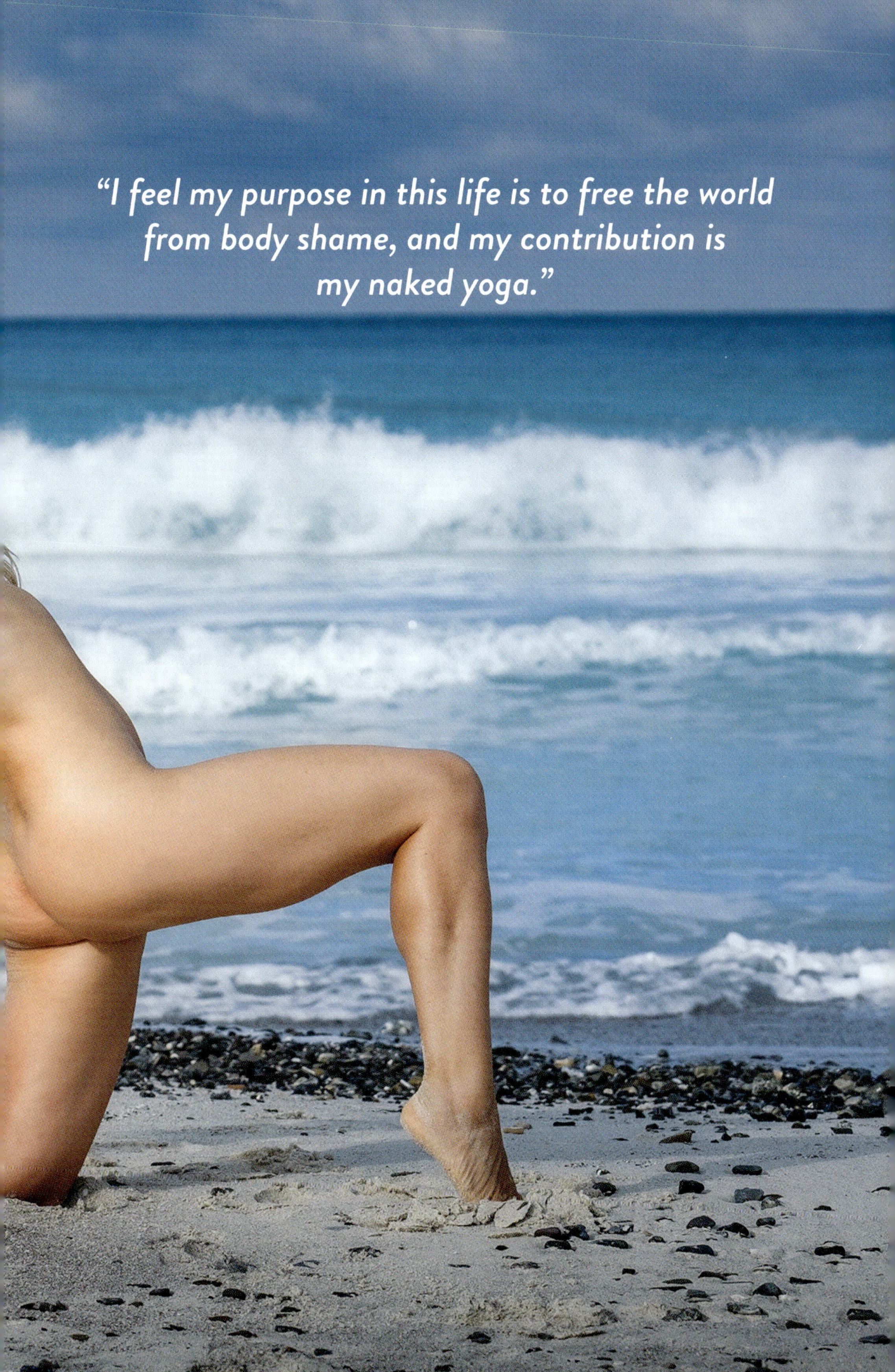
"I feel my purpose in this life is to free the world from body shame, and my contribution is my naked yoga."

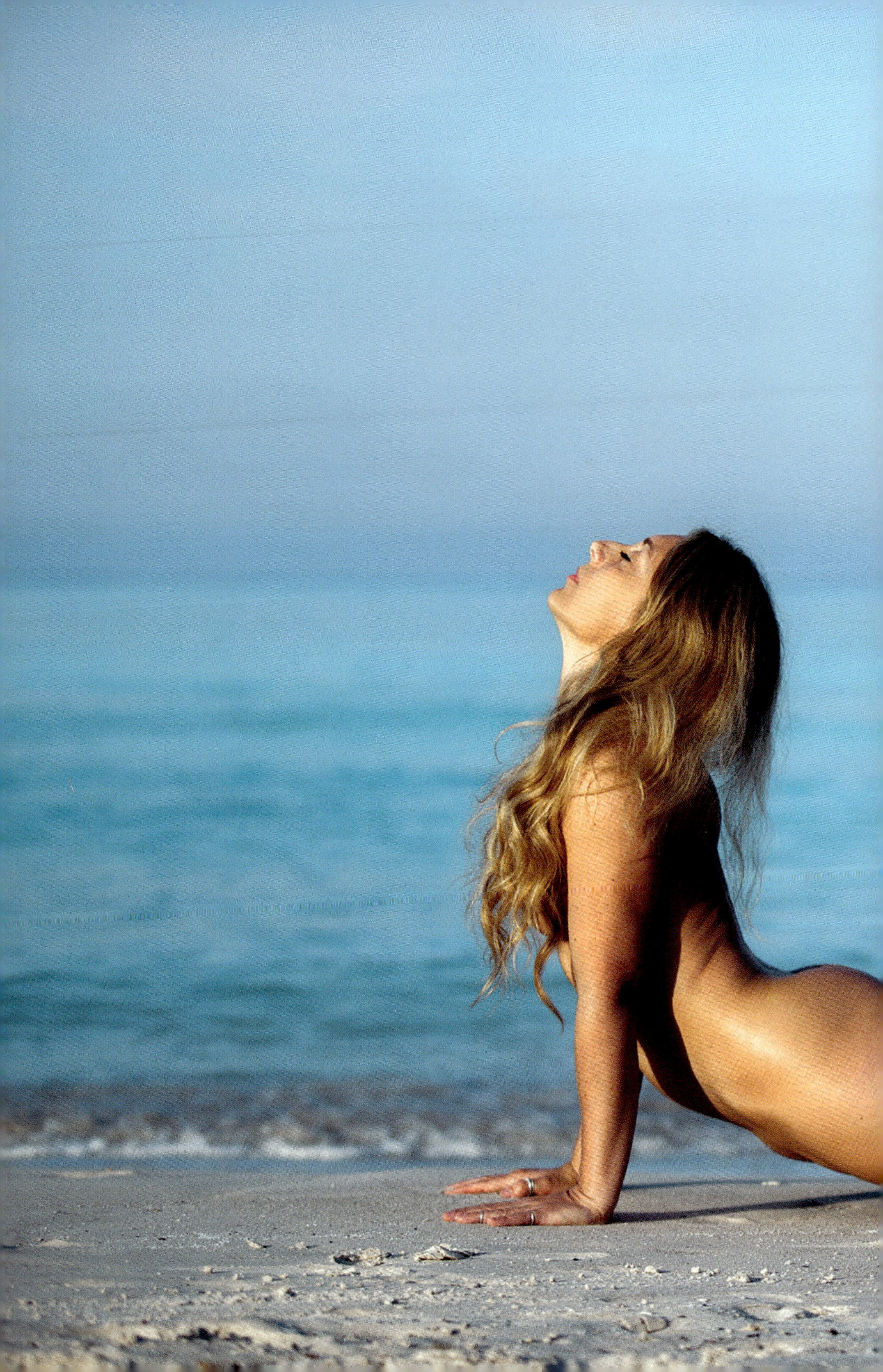

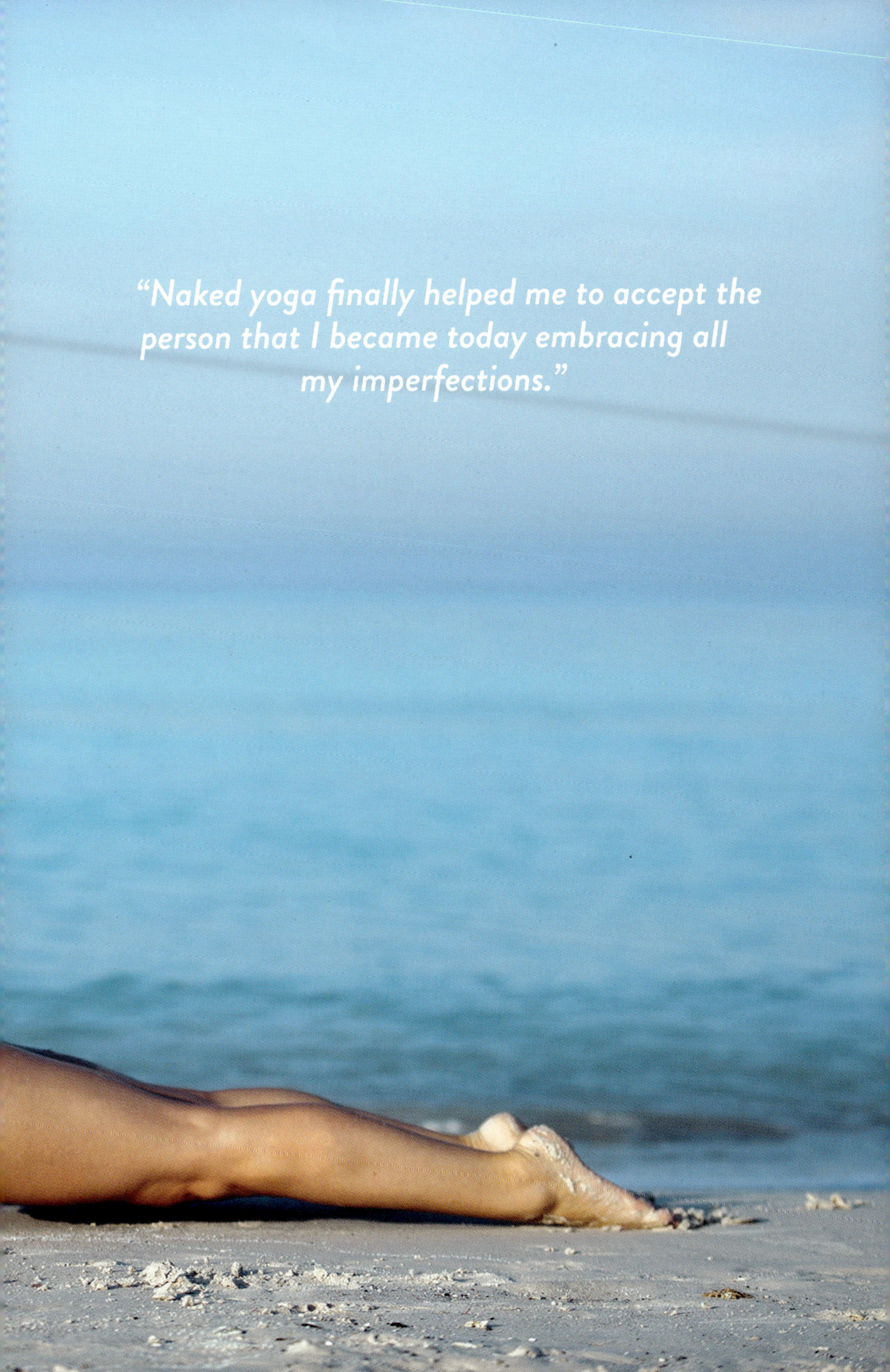
"Naked yoga finally helped me to accept the person that I became today embracing all my imperfections."

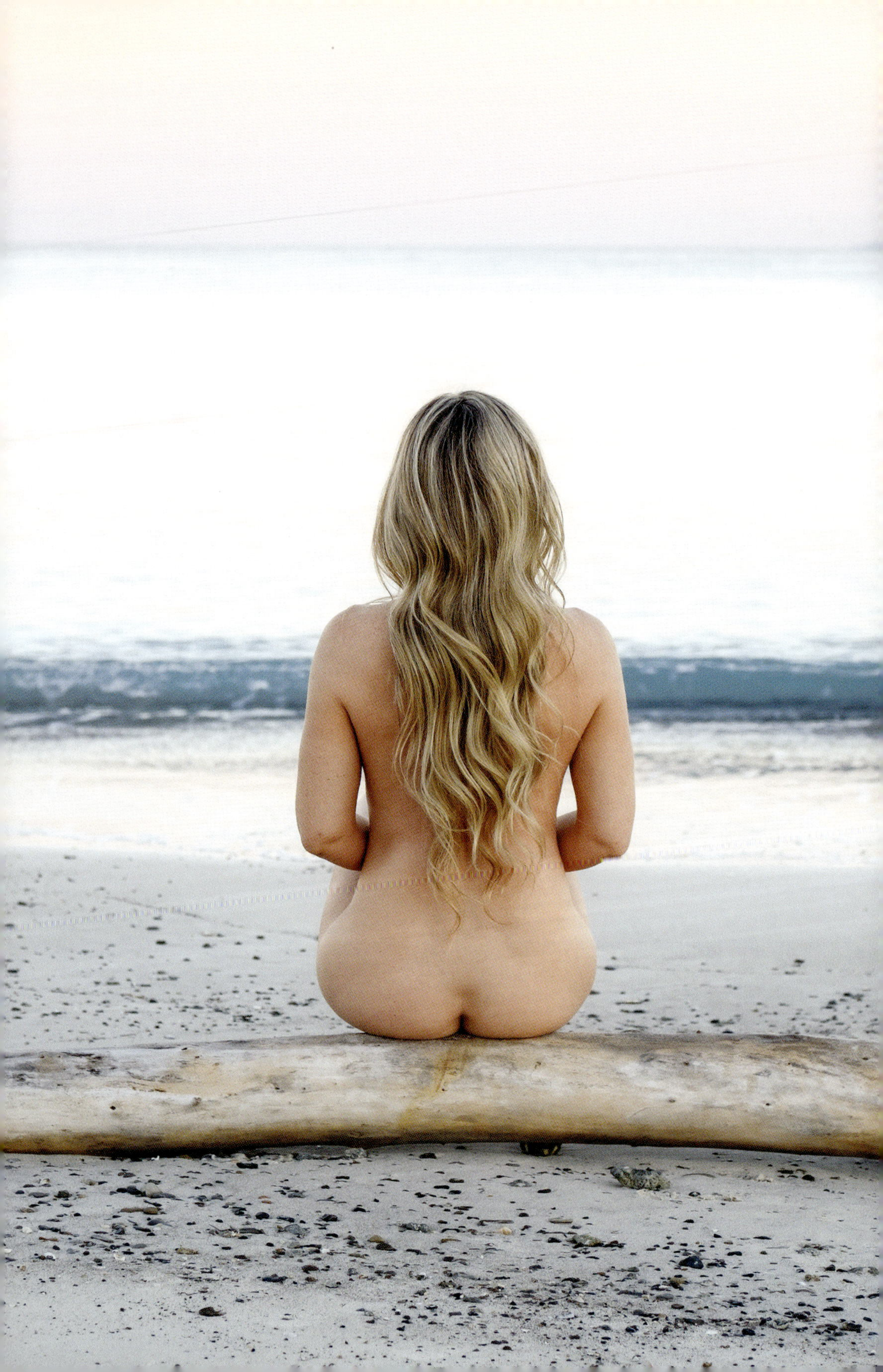

CONTENTS

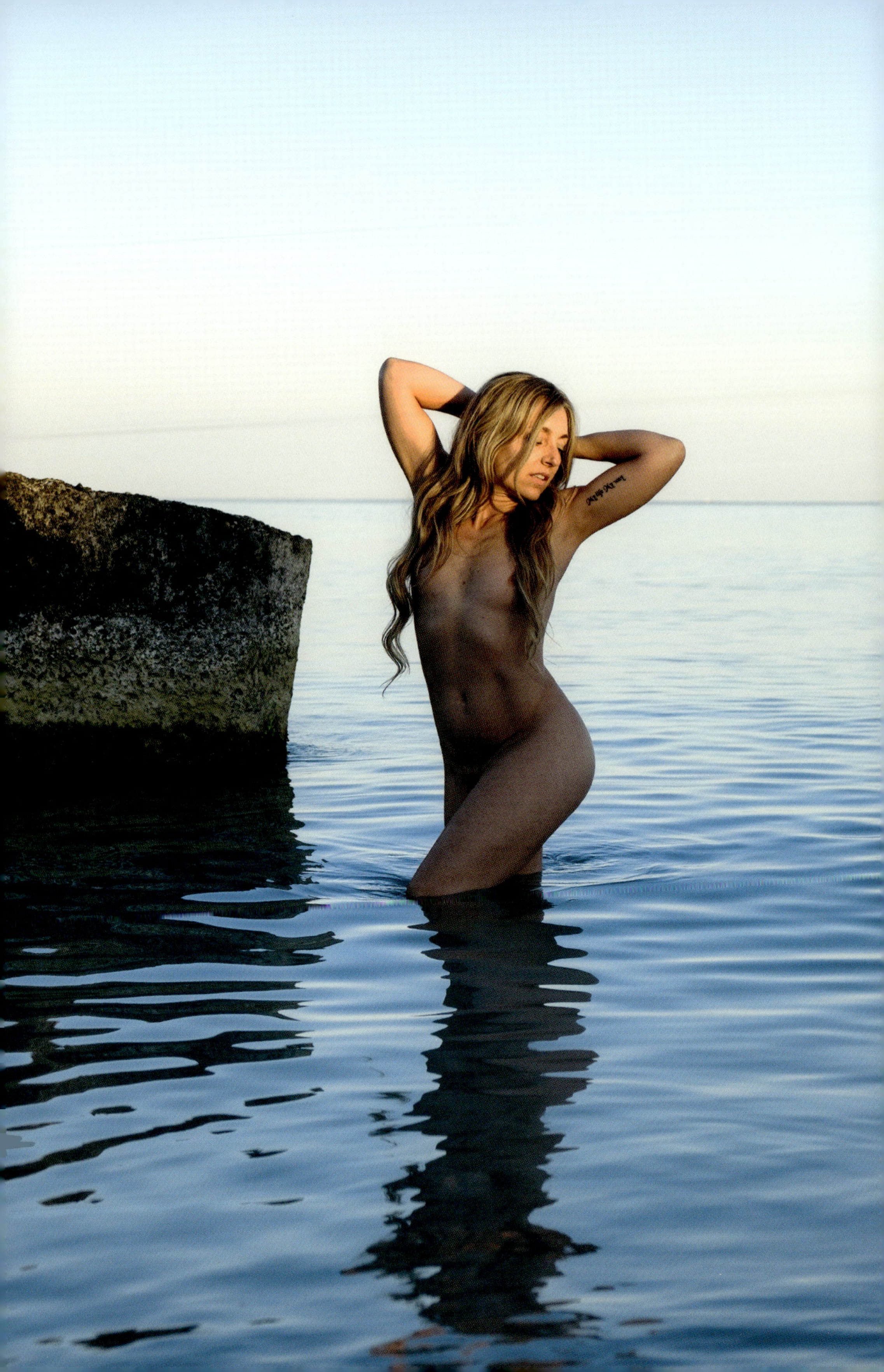

INTRODUCTION

"Nothing is more beautiful than a naked body."
– Yves Saint-Laurent

Every day that I teach yoga, I feel honoured to be in this profession and to have the pleasure to share with my students something that has been so life-changing and empowering for me.

My experience of working in this field for several years has led me to realise the need for advocates of body positivity and for more people generally to challenge outdated notions of shame and embarrassment about the human body.

This book is aimed at those who want to improve their health and fitness in mind, body and spirit. Although some readers will be comfortable with nudity or be practising naturists already, others may have negative attitudes towards their bodies which they wish to overcome, or they may be seeking to achieve a particular physical shape or look. Naked Yoga can free you from the shame and embarrassment of feeling that your body is not good enough, and help you to feel good about being nude in front of others.

Naked Yoga has also helped people suffering from unachievable ideals of bodily perfection, and it can help those suffering from eating disorders or obesity to learn to love their bodies and care for them.

By making a deep and lasting connection with your body, you can learn to listen to its needs and take pleasure in exercising, feeling that you belong in your own skin and that you have a bond with your fellow humans.

In a world where we increasingly spend too much time looking at screens, the simple joy of stretching and bending your body to feel your muscles working, to breathe slowly and calmly, and to set time aside each day for self-care, is more important than ever before.

In this book, I share my own story of rehabilitation from a life-threatening illness and my journey of self-discovery, first of all in taking up yoga and then why I finally decided to teach Naked Yoga.

In Part Two, I aim to build your confidence and fitness through practising yoga naked. By getting used to doing things in the nude, it normalises being naked – by yourself and around others. You will find that many of the ways in which you now judge others no longer seem necessary, and you will start to appreciate new qualities in yourself and other people. By stepping out of your comfort zone you challenge yourself to grow. This leads to greater self-confidence in other areas of your life too, as you are more willing to take on new challenges.

In Part Three, we offer a Beginners' Yoga Guide with advice on how to do simple exercises to get you started with your naked yoga practice in your own home. You will soon find that the idea of wearing yoga pants seems unnatural. Your mind will also grow accustomed to the idea of loving and caring for the body you inhabit and you'll find a new appreciation for walking barefoot. Whether you go on to join a naked yoga class either online or in person, is for you to decide.

Nevertheless, the practice of naked yoga will change your life for the better and help you to understand and appreciate not only your naked body but also your naked self. In Part Four, we hear how it has positively helped some of my students.

Learning yoga is a lifelong journey. I am both a student and a teacher at the same time. I invite you to come on a journey of discovery by reading and following the Beginners' Naked Yoga Guide we have included in this book and realising that, whatever stage in life you are at, naked yoga can only enrich It.

PART ONE

My Journey

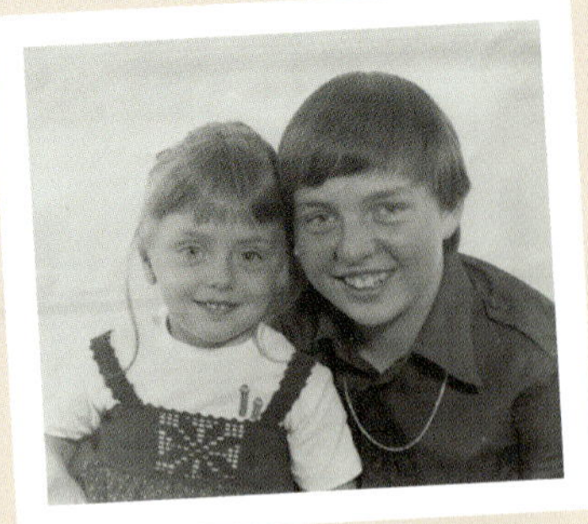

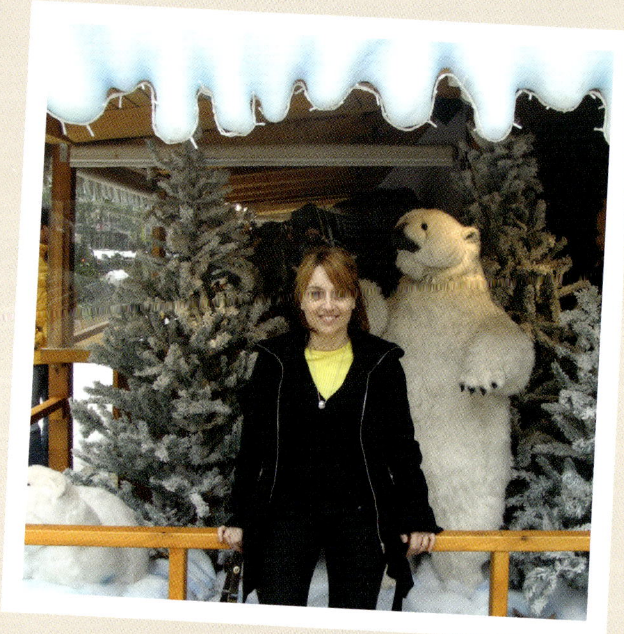

CHAPTER 1

Life Before Cancer

"In order to love who you are, you cannot hate the experiences
that shaped you."
– Andrea Dykstra

Once upon a time, in a small village in Tuscany, Italy, there lived a lost soul who had no idea what to do with her life or what direction to take. My mother did her best to raise me, but my father was the controlling type. I had a very intense love-hate relationship with him which shaped my life.

I had my first taste of body shaming when I was six years old. One morning I woke up and my mother looked at me and began screaming. I was suddenly affected by strabismus, abnormal alignment of the eyes, characterized by a turning inwards or outwards from the nose. This squint was caused officially by paralysis of an eye muscle, and unofficially by a slap in the face.

To correct my squint, I was forced to wear an eye patch and glasses, which inevitably led to my being called "four eyes" at school. Although I was dying of shame and embarrassment, I learned to laugh off those stupid jokes and to redirect the bullies' attention to something else so that they'd leave me in peace. It was two years before I had the necessary eye surgery.

My father's authoritarian behaviour meant that he liked to give orders and expected obedience. Whatever I asked for, the answer was always "No" or "Because I said so". I never had a good relationship with my dad and as much as my mother tried to get us closer she failed in every single attempt. I was 2 years old but her words still run through my head at times: "She's here, happily playing by herself and you come home and make her cry in a matter of seconds." But my father didn't listen. As I grew older, my seething anger made me disruptive at school where I'd often get caught smoking in the toilets or be reprimanded for swearing at the teachers which led to me failing 7th Grade. This behaviour incensed my father, who would often lash out when he got home from work while my mother tried in vain to intervene. I was 12 years old when I exhausted my emotional reserve and attempted suicide.

My brother is ten years older than me, and he still lives at home. He has always needed looking after, and my parents did a great job at making his life much easier. He would often gang up with my father to take his side in family arguments, but if he ever got into trouble, I would go to his defence. Eventually, it got to the point where I often physically fought with my father; he would slap me and push me around. I felt unseen, unheard, and like I wasn't part of the family. An outsider. It wasn't until my teenage years when I would discover physical strength of my own and learn to defend myself, fuelled by the rage I felt towards my father and the unfairness of my situation.

Nothing interested me. I had no passion for anything. There was no debate about my career, as my father and brother both worked for the family real estate business and I was expected to join them. Every detail of my life was arranged by my father. He even insisted on choosing the college where I trained as a structural engineer, ensuring it was local (literally a few hundred metres from where I lived) so he could keep tabs on my movements. After I qualified, I worked for my father for three tiresome years in the hope that I'd get used to the job, maybe even enjoy it one day. Of course, he paid me far less than the going rate.

Next, I trained for the estate agent diploma to be able to sell property, but my father only saw this as another way to exploit me. Instead of paying me the proper commission on my first sale, he gave me only a fraction: 500 euros instead of 5,000. That was the final straw which drove me to leave the family business and take a job working in a shop as a sales assistant. My father went crazy, complaining, "I can't believe my daughter wants to work in a shop handling clothes, when she has such a good career with me! It's a disgrace!" It was time to stop submitting to his tyranny.

I worked as a retail assistant for six months, then I moved to another women's clothes shop where I met the owner who later became my life-long best friend, Antonella. In those two years, I became financially independent of my father. Antonella was a breath of fresh air. She was like the sister I had never had, and we became very close.

Around this time, I met Massimo (not his real name), an attractive older man who was kind and a good listener. I began to feel as though I had a voice and could be heard. The only problem was that he was in a long-standing relationship with another woman. He actually helped me to understand a little bit more about my relationship with my father and we became close friends. This intimacy progressed into a sexual relationship which was exciting, partially because it was conducted in secret behind the back of his long-term partner, heightened by the sense of it being forbidden.

While I was working with Antonella, I had the time to reflect on my life and I decided to quit my job and go back to university. I asked my father for financial support but, unsurprisingly, he refused to help. "I don't understand why you should go back to study, or why you want to go to university? It's pointless," he said.

I decided to study Spanish and English to become a translator and interpreter and follow my dream of travelling. I juggled working part-time in three different jobs to support my studies. It was an expensive course, and I had to travel by train to the university about 40 miles away. The summer before graduating, I decided to move to Spain for a few months to gain a deeper understanding of the Spanish language. My father thought this was a ridiculous idea, but I went anyway as I was determined to learn as much Spanish as I could.

I moved to Santander, and it was wonderful to learn a new culture and be free to meet new people and try new experiences. One day, Massimo surprised me with an unexpected visit. I don't know how he found me as I hadn't given him my address, but I was pleased to see him and we spent a fun week together, travelling around. We drank cañas, ate paella and pinchos and had the most wonderful time. Being so far away from everybody we knew back home, we could relax and enjoy each other's company. After that, we spent two hours talking every day on the phone and so I went back to Italy at the end of the summer before the start of my last year at the university expecting our relationship to blossom.

When Massimo put a ring on my finger, I was thrilled, believing he was serious about our future together, but after several months he still couldn't bring himself to leave his long-term partner. He wouldn't let me tell my best friend Antonella about our relationship either and after three years of being controlled by him, I had to face the truth that this relationship was going nowhere. It seemed to be an echo of my father's behaviour, leaving me with feelings of being used and unloved. My friend, Antonella, supported me through the whole sorry saga. With the help of a psychotherapist, and a lot of soul-searching, I eventually broke up with Massimo. I finally understood that being controlled and manipulated by a man wasn't the same as being loved.

Right after graduating, one of my university tutors offered me a job. The work involved being a guide and interpreter for Spanish tourists on cruises around the Mediterranean visiting Pisa and Florence on day trips. It was a very exciting opportunity, and I accepted this new challenge.

When the summer season was over, I decided to move to London for a couple of months to improve my English so I could work with American and English tourists as well. I wasn't excited about starting again from scratch, having to look for a new place to live and a new job, but I knew it was the right step to take for my career. However, when I got to London, I decided to take my career in a completely different direction. I suddenly felt I was free for the first time in my life – and it felt wonderful.

I found a job in two days in a shop with a Spanish company. I met beautiful people from different walks of life. I began to have fun, and I was finally able to be fully myself. Once I had experienced this feeling of freedom, I couldn't face going home again. One month led to another and, as I began to enjoy my independence, I had no desire to go back to live in a place where I would be forced to be home by midnight. I'd become something of a joke to my friends back in Italy. They were used to going out partying or clubbing until 6am in the morning, and slowly they had stopped inviting me out.

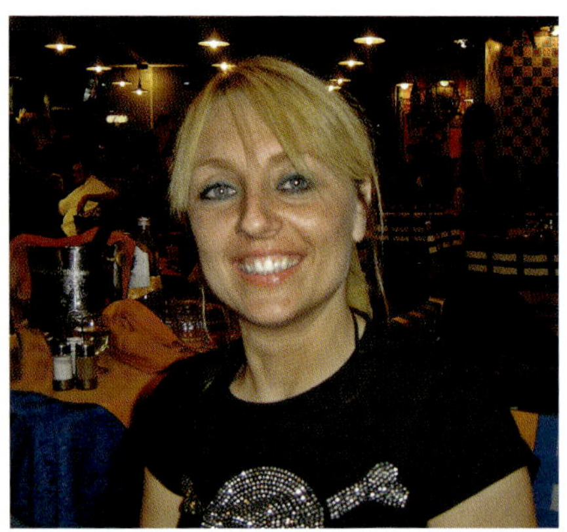

I soon got offered a job as a supervisor for another Spanish company. I loved the Spanish language, and I found myself being part of a nice big family. This new job gave me the knowledge and confidence to later run a flagship store in Regent Street. It was a lot of responsibility and I was sick, but I didn't know it yet.

Each year, when I went back to Italy for a short visit, I would see my doctor to have a smear test and breast cancer check-up. They had always come back negative. I was in a relationship in London and I noticed that whenever my boyfriend and I had sex, I would bleed a little. As it wasn't painful, it was a while before I went to see my doctor in London. Having recently started taking the pill, I thought it might have something to do with that, that maybe my body needed some more time to adapt to this new hormonal storm. My GP ran some blood tests and when the results came back with abnormal blood cells, he asked me to redo the tests for confirmation. Then I was sent to a hospital for a cervical biopsy.

Having the biopsy was a traumatic experience. The embarrassment I felt at having medical staff examining my cervix was nothing compared to the invasiveness of the procedure without even an anaesthetic. It triggered a huge panic attack and I started to hyperventilate. I went rigid with fright, my arms, hands and mouth paralysed, I thought I was going to die.

The results of the biopsy came back quickly. I didn't know then that my life was about to change forever.

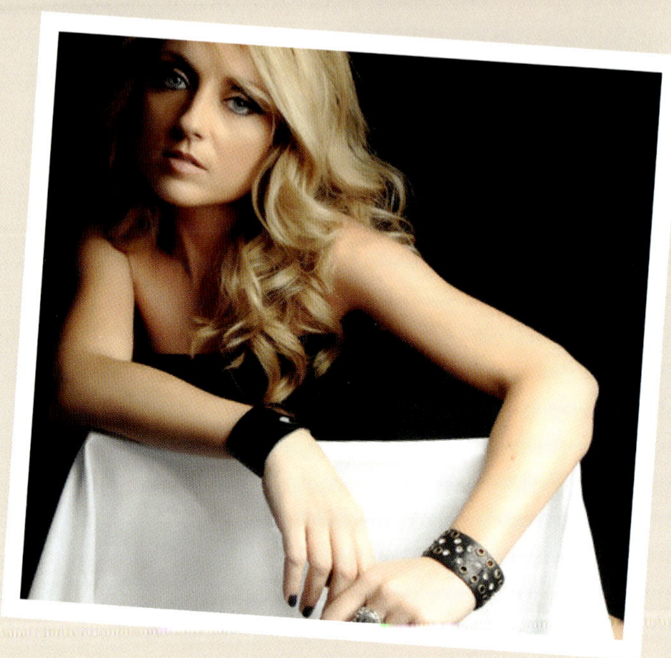

CHAPTER 2

Facing The Big 'C'

"It takes one moment to hate who you are, and a lifetime to remember how to love yourself again. This is the most important war."
– Erin Van Vuren

A week after the awful experience of the biopsy, I went back to the hospital and they handed me a piece of paper that told me I had stage-3 cervical cancer. I went into shock. I couldn't feel anything. The whole world seemed to stop.

As the doctor explained to me that I would need a major operation, it seemed as though this was happening to somebody else. It didn't seem possible that I could be suffering from such a serious illness. I had planned to go through with the surgery without telling my parents, but as the seriousness of the situation began to sink in, I felt desperately alone.

I called my brother and he started to cry. He couldn't believe it was happening to me. He was very scared and wanted to tell my parents straight away but I said that I would tell them myself when I was ready to. What was the point of telling them? I thought that my father would only make me feel guilty about contracting such an illness, as if I deserved it for living my life as an independent woman.

Finally, I called my best friend Antonella and although she was surprised, she was very grounded and said, "We will get through this together, let's take one step at the time" She gave me love and support unconditionally – which helped me come to terms with the diagnosis. Her friendship was invaluable.

The next time I had to go in for an internal examination, I asked the anaesthetist to give me a general anaesthetic so that I didn't have another panic attack. As I was unconscious for the examination and test, I didn't realise until I woke up that something had gone wrong and I found myself covered in blood. As soon as I called out for a nurse and they saw that I was haemorrhaging, it felt like panic stations and I was rushed back into the operating room. By then I was screaming at them not to touch me again without another anaesthesia, and they had to sedate me to calm me down. When I woke up the second time it was all over – for now!

Of course, when I did tell my parents, they tried to talk me into going back to Italy for medical treatment. They began asking around for recommendations of good local cancer specialists. My mother told me that one of our neighbours in Italy also had cervical cancer. She had heard of all the gruesome procedures from our neighbour and was terrified that her daughter would be going through the same things.

My father kept trying to push me to go back to Italy, but I refused. I felt safe and supported by the NHS staff in London. I had met really wonderful nurses and doctors and I trusted them to take good care of me. My main operation date was set for 14th April, and my parents arrived in London two days before the operation.

Waiting to go into the operation room, I couldn't stop thinking about Massimo, I missed him and I missed his words. "Don't worry, I will take care of you," as he used to say to me. So, I had the *brilliant* idea to call him for some support. We hadn't spoken for five years, so I changed my phone settings to call him with a private number.

"Hi, do you remember me?" I said.

"Of course, I do. How could I ever forget about you?"

Almost immediately, all of my expectations dropped as he coolly suggested that we might meet up for a coffee when I next visited Italy. I don't know what I had expected, but I felt really let down once again.

This caused me to reflect on the relationship and how it had made me feel undervalued and unloved. In hindsight, I recognized that it had produced the same feelings I'd had in my relationship with my father. A sense of absolute worthlessness.

I'd always felt guilty about being in a relationship with him because he was involved in another relationship. Had my sense of worthlessness triggered the cancer? I was thrashing around, searching for answers. I kept thinking about how this cancer was linked to the most intimate part of my body, the part in charge of creation. What did I know or feel about my body? Was I comfortable with the idea of my own sexuality? It seemed that if I loved my body and enjoyed myself as a sexually liberated woman, then I felt guilty. Whereas if I hated my body and felt ashamed of it, which I did most of the time, it was damaging to me both physically and psychologically. I needed to break out of this vicious circle of guilt and shame.

I went into the operation room and I counted one… two… then I was out. The sensation as the aesthetic started to work was incredible. I was floating on high. At peace with everything. I wasn't scared despite what I had gone through for my first operation. I just accepted it all as a necessary course of action for me to go on living. The operation was supposed to last for about three hours, but due to complications it ended up lasting seven hours.

When I eventually came around from the anaesthetic, I was surprised to find bandages all over my body. As well as my cervix, six of my lymph nodes had been contaminated by cancer cells, and to prevent it spreading further, they had decided to remove all of them.

Once I had fully gained consciousness, I had this huge urge to get up and go to the toilet, which wasn't possible as I was attached to so many machines. A nurse introduced me to 'my bag'. I discovered that I was attached to a colostomy bag by a drainage tube. Initially, this completely phased me but after a while I got used to the bag and called it my Louis Vuitton bag.

The day after the operation, the nurses started my rehabilitation. I thought they were kidding as I felt so much pain, but they insisted that I try to walk a little each day as this would help me heal faster. I would walk a few steps with two nurses holding me up and each day I went a little further around the ward, along with my bag. At this point, I didn't care how I looked and often ended up laughing a lot with the nurses – being alive was enough.

On the fifth day, the nurses removed my Louis Vuitton bag – the tube was long – I had thought about this moment since I was told that I was going to have this operation. The idea of having a tube removed from my body while being fully awake made me feel so nauscous. I couldn't talk or breathe. I could hear my heartbeat pounding like crazy, inhaling and exhaling until the tube was gone.

After a week of recovery, I was allowed home. At the time, I had a room in a shared apartment with my landlady. As I needed help around the clock for the first three months after the operation, my mother offered to stay with me. She was a rock – unlike my father who couldn't handle it at all and went back to Italy to take care of the family business, soon after I came out of hospital. My landlady wasn't exactly supportive either and despite the fact that my room was big enough for myself and my mother to stay in, she made me rent another room for my mother to put her clothes in.

During those first three months I stayed in bed or visited the hospital for chemotherapy and radiotherapy. I felt so tired all the time that I couldn't rouse myself to get out of bed – everything felt as if it was too much effort.

I had so many negative thoughts towards myself that I believed I had created this illness because of my own sense of worthlessness in my relationship with Massimo. I basically blamed myself for becoming sick and felt as if cancer was a natural step to go through after so much negativity.

The radiotherapy brought with it another major dilemma too. I would have to choose between keeping my fertility or saving my life.

CHAPTER 3

A Life-Changing Decision

"Your body is the piece of the universe you've been given, the place where love and joy and grief happen, where happiness unfolds. Do you really want to keep believing that it's a horrible, ugly, lumpy thing? Do you really want to keep punching yourself like that?"
– Geneen Roth

While I had been recovering from the biopsy and coming to terms with my cancer diagnosis, another dilemma had presented itself. The doctor gently explained to me that the radiotherapy treatment would render me infertile. I had to make a choice quickly between saving my eggs – or saving my life – the decision was that black and white.

Although I thought of freezing my eggs before the operation, the doctor told me that the procedure to remove them, would increase the chance of touching one of the cancerous cells and spreading the cancer beyond control. He also explained that even if they successfully managed to extract an egg without any damage, there was only a 20 per cent chance of future IVF being successful.

To be honest, I'd never been a maternal person, and children were not on the horizon for me any time soon. However, the thought of never being able to have a child was devastating. It seemed that the option to become a mother was being taken away from me before I had ever seriously considered it.

Somehow I had never pictured myself getting married or settling down with a husband and two kids. Although I was in a relationship at the time, I knew that my boyfriend wasn't the person I wanted to share my life with. I discussed the options with him and also with my mother and my best friend Antonella, but in the end, it became clear that I had to make a choice between losing my fertility or losing my life.

Reluctantly, I chose to give up on any chance of having a child. Only later would I realise what a huge emotional impact that would have on me. Once the operation was over and the treatments started, I knew there was no going back. It was at that point that I really hit a low as I suddenly felt that no one would ever love me or want a long-term relationship with me as I would never be able to conceive a child. Who would ever want to share his life with a dry empty sack?

The endless trips to the hospital were taking their toll on my mind and body too. The side effects made me very weak, and I had to put all my energy into getting through the different treatments, simply surviving one day at a time. The chemotherapy gave me constipation and I took medication to counter the nausea and vomiting which are common side effects. On top of this, the radiotherapy gave me diarrhoea and made my skin very sore and dry in the treatment area. My body was reeling from being subjected to both these treatments at the same time. The next piece of shocking news came when the doctor advised me to prepare for the onset of early menopause and that I had to face the prospect of rapidly aging twenty years before my time.

As if that news was not hard enough to deal with, the medical advice that I would also need to insert a plastic contraption, called a dilator, into my vagina on a daily basis to prevent shrinkage was an additional unavoidable torment. Although they start you off with a small dilator, around the size of a tampon, even that was excruciatingly painful as the abrasions caused by the radiation treatment produced scar tissue inside the vagina. The dilator helped to stretch my vagina and soften the scar tissue but every time I used one, it caused bleeding, adding to my distress and worry. What else could this disease throw at me?

During this time of ongoing treatments, I felt as if I had become a patient rather than a person. The medical profession had taken over my life completely and I had to follow instructions and be compliant – just the way I had been as a child back in Italy.

It was important to eat before the chemotherapy as, after only five minutes of receiving toxic chemicals into my body, my stomach couldn't take even the smallest amount of food. All the lights on the machines used to blur as I tried really hard to go somewhere else and not to be present in the room. I didn't form a 'chat club' with the other patients there, even though I would often be in the room with the same people for hours on end. Each of us was a kind of island as we tried to block out the noise of the machines and deal with the emotional roller-coaster of what was happening to us and the dangers we still faced.

I did get to know my radiotherapy nurse very well, whose name was Sandra, the kindest 'big mama'. The medical staff marked black dots on my body, to enable the radiology teams to pinpoint the right areas for treatment. I still have these little tattoos.

Some people lost their hair and wore head coverings, others didn't bother. Some were so thin that they looked as if they were starving, a few looked pale and deathlike, while others looked so robust and healthy, it would have been hard to tell they were sick at all. A handful of people were there for the first time, others were back for the second or third time as they battled the disease. It was an awful thought that I might have to face this disease again when I was older. It had already left me feeling like an old woman inside, and I was young. I wondered how they managed to cope physically and mentally going through the whole business over and over again. When the treatment was finally over, my mother would help me drag myself home on the bus. I couldn't have gone through it without her – she was my safety net.

Of course, I was offered counselling support as I struggled with shame and guilt over getting cancer in such an intimate part of my body. It was a revelation to learn that cervical cancer is often the result of being infected with HPV (Human Papillomavirus Infection), of which there are over a hundred different types. The virus is often transmitted during sex without either party being aware of it. You can avoid infection by having a vaccination to protect you against HPV.

The US Center for Disease Control and Prevention recommends that pre-teens be vaccinated before any likely exposure to sexually transmitted strains of HPV. It's important to get regular tests to check for abnormalities too.

Counselling helped me to see that I had to stop blaming myself for my illness. My self-loathing was harmful to my recovery. I had to start loving myself and begin to accept myself as I am now. I had to stop and listen to my body in a way that I had never listened to it before. I had to work out what I really wanted for my life and go towards that future.

I couldn't save my eggs, but I had to save Doria.

CHAPTER 4

Finding Doria

*"You're going to be in your own skin until you die. That's a while.
You might as well get comfortable in it."*
(Unknown)

With all the time I spent in hospital I had hours to reflect on my past and to question why I had become ill and what I was doing with my life. Although I have never been religious, there were times when I was so scared that I prayed for everything to be all right. I even found myself wondering if God was punishing me for my past misdeeds such as having an affair with a man who was already in a committed relationship.

I was living in an alternative reality, a kind of limbo where my life was on hold while I was focused on getting better and nothing else. Hopes and dreams of my previous life had to be abandoned as I began to accept that the old normal was never going to be there for me again. Dealing with the fatigue and the loss of appetite meant that I had little energy to imagine a different kind of life for myself. I was too busy grieving for my old life. It was when I was at my lowest point that I felt truly alone and frightened. I had to reach down into the well of my being and find the inner strength to carry on fighting for my life. It was then that the person I am now began to emerge.

As a teenager I had been bulimic, vomiting up food to try and maintain an impossibly low weight. At 25, I only weighed 40 kilos, but even that wasn't thin enough. I always wanted to have the perfect body, and constantly failed to achieve this. My drive for perfection, to be the golden girl for my father and win his approval, had only left me feeling worthless and ashamed.

Now these feelings of shame and worthlessness were magnified. I was a youngish woman going through an early menopause, and when I tried to resume a physical relationship with my boyfriend, I found sex painful and difficult.

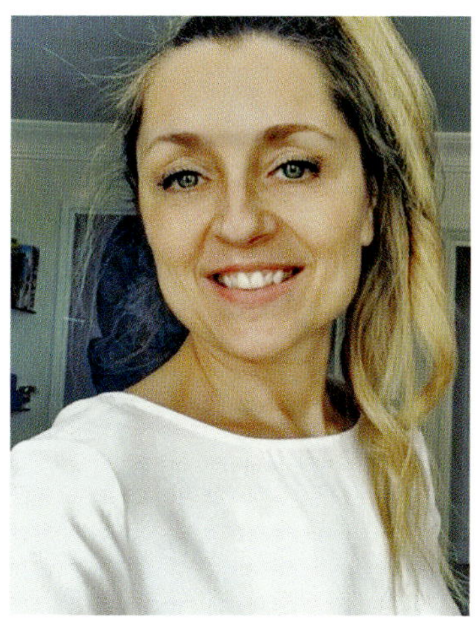

When I finally went back to Italy for a rest, my father added to my distress by saying things like "Who would marry you now?" or "When will you have any children?" despite the fact that he knew it was impossible. Most of my friends in the village back in Tuscany were married by then and quite a few had children so being back there only accentuated the fact that I was never going to fit in with that community. I felt suffocated and knew I had to escape as soon as I was well enough.

I couldn't help imagining awful images of my body being cut, and the swollen parts of myself were a visual reminder. I kept thinking: this is it now. I have this body and I can't change it. I can't get in shape by going to the gym. When I looked in the mirror I felt totally disconnected from my body. Who was that person I could see? It didn't feel like me anymore.

While my fear of being judged as someone broken and incomplete increased, I had a desperate need to feel loved. Fortunately, I was offered counselling to deal with my emotional turmoil and through talking about my experiences I came to recognize that there was a part of me that had always been longing terribly for love and acceptance and always feeling lost and empty.

Whereas I had always looked to others to fill this void in me, now I was going to have to find a way to complete myself. I had to begin to take care of myself and so I was looking for ways to heal and help my recovery, both mentally and physically. One of the nurses at the Macmillan Cancer Support Centre suggested that I try going to one of the yoga classes which they offered. That was the beginning.

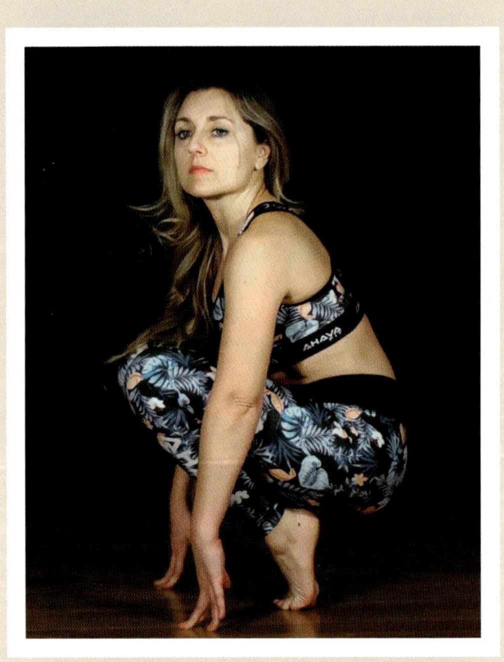

CHAPTER 5

Discovering Yoga

The first time I tried yoga, it was in a Macmillan Cancer Support Centre. It was a very gentle practice as I was with other students affected by cancer. During the class, it was all so strange that I kept looking around and checking other people's expressions, but I couldn't catch any, as they were busy enjoying the session. The movements were new and didn't make any sense. It was confusing, and I couldn't find the connection. At the end of the class, I left the room doubtful it had done any good. I couldn't understand what the attraction was for the other women, but I decided to go back again the following week.

One week later, on a Tuesday, I found myself looking for an answer, sitting down in a crossed-legged position like an old yogi, on the same spot as the previous week. At the end of the class, when I opened my eyes after the deep breathing of *Shavasana* (final relaxation) and I was blessed with the experience of a yoga high, I had my answer – the feeling was exquisite. Everything in my body was alive. It felt wonderful to physically notice my toes, to feel the weight of my body sinking into the ground, to imagine my imprint on the earth as I let go.

I went back to yoga classes again and again and noticed that my spirits were lifting, and I began to feel better about myself too – lighter. Once I'd finished at the Macmillan Cancer Support Centre, I knew that I had to continue going to yoga. First, I tried doing yoga in a health club, which turned out to be a lot more challenging than the classes on offer for people recovering from cancer, but I persisted, and eventually, I was going most days to different clubs in London and I took advantage of the introductory offers of half the yoga studios in London. My days all had the same schedule: work and yoga, work and yoga, work and yoga. I was in love with this discipline, and more importantly I was noticing my body getting stronger every day. I was slowly feeling 'normal' again.

In the meantime, I was promoted to become a store manager at one of the four major shops that dominate Oxford Circus. I thought I had made it. However, the pressure of working long hours, leaving home before 7am and getting home at 11pm, was taking its toll. It looked glamorous to be in the fashion industry, in one of the top shops in London, but in reality, it was exhausting. My life was a mess: I was managing thirty people and my job was incredibly stressful, and suddenly I started to bleed again. I got so scared that I decided to leave my job and move back to Italy for a few months for a complete health check-up. Once there, I went through a very bad depression.

Back at home with my parents, I was spending my days watching TV and eating crisps on the sofa. The doctor confirmed the bleeding was only the body still adjusting after the treatments, which was a great relief. My father was pressuring me to take charge of the family business. Once again, I found myself lost and unhappy and with the responsibility of running the family business which was something I had never wanted to do. My father's harassment made it worse. I went to see a therapist again, the same woman I had seen many years previously. She helped me to understand that this was *my* life, and I was in charge of it.

A few weeks later I packed everything up and went back to London. It was hard for my father to accept my decision and he tried everything to persuade me to stay. Back in London, I decided not to return to working in retail. Unemployed, crashing on the sofa at my friend's place, I began looking for an office job. My goal was to find a boring job with weekends off. After spending so many Christmases and bank holidays working on the shop floor, I desperately wanted some stability and structure in my life.

During this time, I was exploring various forms of yoga in London. I used my new-found energy to change my career and find a nice place to live. I moved away from the stressful world of the retail fashion industry into the world of people and communications in Human Resources. Once I was working again, I felt I had a future and I enjoyed working in a team and making new friends.

Finally, my life was getting back on track and it occurred to me that it would be amazing to learn more about the philosophy behind yoga. The practice itself didn't fulfil me in the same way anymore. Was I thinking of becoming a yoga teacher? "Oh no! No way," it was just to enrich my knowledge as a student.

I asked my teachers where they had done their certifications, trying to memorise every single word coming out of their mouths. They talked about different styles of yoga which I had never heard of before, and I knew I had more to learn. Google search helped me to discover the many routes available to getting a yoga teacher diploma. I could choose to attend a weekend course spread over six months or a one-month intensive course to become a yoga teacher in only twenty-six days. Scary... and exciting.

It seemed that India was definitely the home of yoga, and I was dying to visit this beautiful country. To choose from all the courses offered around the world, I first needed to decide what style of yoga I wanted to train in. I became obsessed. I began experimenting in the different yoga studios in London, trying out different teachers and styles of yoga. Every day I learned something new; it was exciting and sometimes frustrating as some students in the class had a very advanced practice, beyond anything I could achieve at the time.

Many hours spent sweating on a yoga mat later, I came to the conclusion that Ashtanga yoga was definitely my match. It is a precise and physically demanding practice. It takes on average ninety minutes to complete the Full Primary Series – longer than most yoga or fitness classes. The tradition asks you to practise six days a week, which is a difficult commitment to make. Discipline was the key. Ashtanga yoga became the focus of my day and started to become the centre of my life.

Nothing could distract me from it – when I had my yoga class, nothing else mattered. Friends could wait, life could wait, yoga came first. I lived, breathed, dreamed, drank, ate, slept and talked only about yoga. It was my everything. It made such a huge impact on my life that I couldn't afford to go back to that dark place where I had been. Unmotivated and lost. I finally felt my body had come alive after such a long time. I was driven, inspired, curious and finally healing.

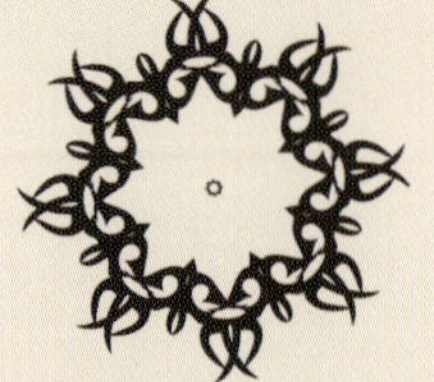

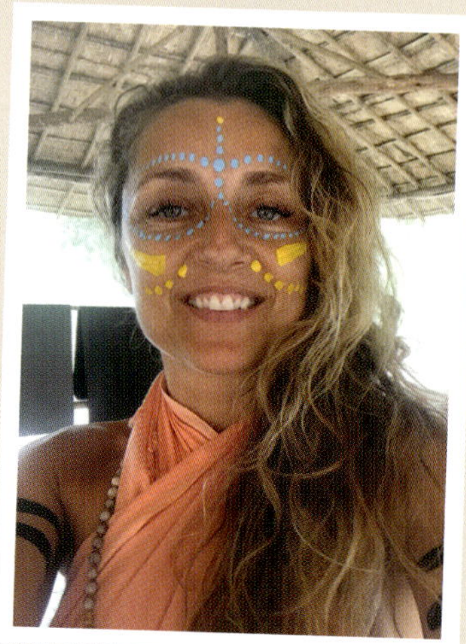

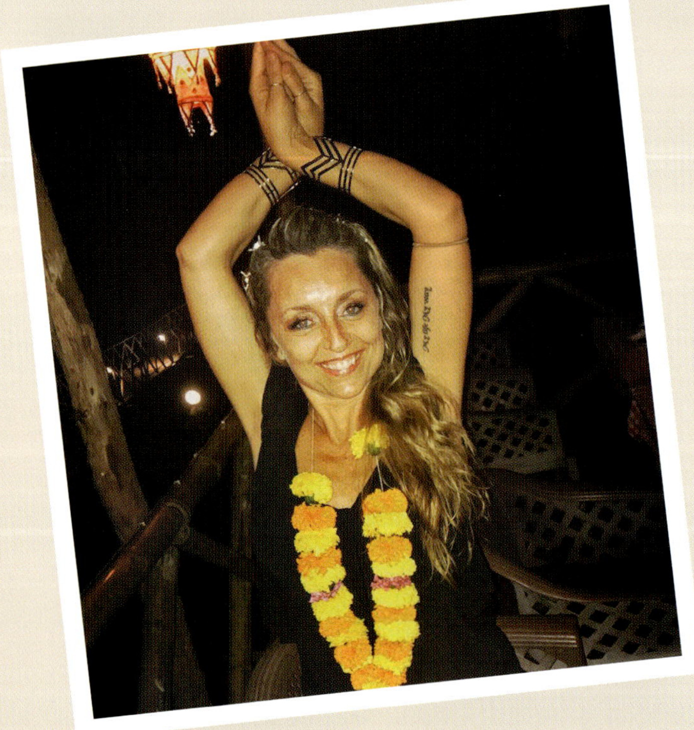

CHAPTER 6

Journey To India

*"The healer you have been looking for is your own courage to know
and love yourself completely."*
– Yung Pueblo

By 2014, I was spending almost every evening going to yoga classes. The practice of yoga had an energizing effect on me, and it offered me a new way of being in the world as it also calmed my troubled mind. I knew I had to devote time to healing myself and living in a way that was more in harmony with my spirit. I found myself wanting to learn more and delve deeper into the philosophy behind this ancient practice.

I found a course in India that taught the style of yoga that I particularly liked – Ashtanga yoga – which is a more energetic style in which you learn to synchronize your breath with the movements. It was based on the traditional poses and I spent weeks arguing with myself about whether I really wanted to go or not, coming up with excuses like: "You can't take a month off" or "You can't afford to go" and even "India is a long way away and a dangerous place for a western woman travelling by herself." Luckily, I had a very good friend at work, Pilar, and she encouraged me to go. I don't think I would have taken the plunge to go to India without her giving me a gentle push. The tipping point was when she said, "Losing £800 might change your life – and if you never go you will never know."

I plucked up my courage and went to see my HR manager and asked for six weeks off work so I could attend the course and have a few days looking around India. To my surprise, they were happy to help and interested in what I was doing. I bought my air tickets and put my inner critic back in its box – at least for a while.

I had chosen a course for trainee yoga teachers which offered 200 hours of training. At that point, I actually had no intention of practising as a yoga teacher – I wanted to get deeper into yoga both physically and spiritually and to understand the history and philosophy behind it.

When I first arrived in New Delhi, I was truly shocked by the chaos. The sight of so many men at the airport, with no women around was daunting. India was a revelation: all the sights and smells, the vibrant drama of the streets, and the teeming throngs of people. The Taj Mahal was the highlight of my trip. I stood in front of the monument for two hours, transfixed by its sheer beauty and majesty.

I wanted to experience the real India, so I travelled by local transport, and what an adventure! Twelve-hour trips on a night bus, train journeys at night, in which people stared at me as if I was an alien from Mars. I quickly understood it was important to appear to be a married woman, so I moved my ring from the thumb to the ring finger of my left hand. Some of my fellow travellers were curious, asking lots of questions or wanting me to take a picture with them, especially if they had kids.

I witnessed a man under a bridge piercing a boy's nose with a rusty nail; poor kids, naked, playing on top of a mountain of stinking rubbish; a meat market with the worst imaginable smell, the meat lying outside in 40 degree heat with stray dogs and crows eating the entrails of the animals on the ground. This was the India I wanted to see. Not the lavish India of a five-star hotel.

It was exciting to be travelling as this was one of the things I'd always wanted to do. The training centre in Goa was fairly basic with simple beds and vegetarian food. People had come from all over the world to attend the course and most were committed yogis, who lived and breathed yoga. The course itself was extremely hard core – with yoga training for twelve hours per day, six and a half days per week. It was both wonderful and exhausting. Every day I felt myself getting more and more in touch with myself as a person. Not the self-loathing Doria that I had been in hospital – but a new Doria whom I had never really known before.

I met some wonderful souls in training, and together we grew and connected on a deeper level. We cried, got stronger, stepped out of our comfort zones, and communicated our feelings and thoughts – all together. Yoga wasn't just *asanas;* it was life. It's here where I met Emma, a beautiful lost soul, and we became inseparable.

She made this training an adventure, filled with fun. We complimented each other: I was the masculine energy, she was the feminine energy, she was Ida, I was Pingala, we still are.

Learning about the chakras was a revelation, understanding that everything is connected – the way you are, the way you react – it's all linked to your past and to your parents and their behaviours. Many tears flowed during this lecture and some people had to leave the room as they felt too broken to go on. All of us were dealing with past trauma and the shared understanding of our suffering bound us together.

The day of the final exam came, and I had to run a class in front of a panel of teachers for a group which included one of the most difficult students. I was sure this student didn't like me, and I had no confidence that they would do what I asked. In the end, using some of my old management skills and gentle persuasion, along with sharing how to do the various moves in a nonthreatening way, I managed to get this student to comply and I passed the exam with a distinction. I was now a qualified yoga teacher – not that I had any intention of teaching back then nor the confidence to do so – but that would come later.

Once I got back to London, people at the various yoga studios were curious about my experience. Going to India had given me a different view of the world and of my place within it. I felt connected to an ancient wisdom going back millennia. When I told them I had qualified as a teacher, they asked me to teach some classes. My inner critic kept saying, "You aren't really good enough – what do you know?" But one day, Jonelle, one of my friends from the training who had already started to teach, said she urgently needed a cover for her class, so could I do it as a favour?

My initial reaction was to say, "No, I'm not ready." The prospect of teaching a yoga class filled me with dread. Did I even remember the sequence? I couldn't do it. But my friend told me that she had already confirmed my details with the yoga studio owner. I couldn't believe it. I was furious, I felt sick to my stomach. Reluctantly, I agreed. I couldn't think about anything else for a week. I couldn't talk about it; I was too nervous. Within days I was walking into my first yoga class as a teacher, terrified.

The class seemed to go well, and I was elated. It was only when I got home and reflected on the experience that I realised I actually loved teaching yoga. It came as something of a surprise as I had a well-paid job I enjoyed doing and I wasn't looking to change my career again. As I continued to teach yoga over those first few weeks, my confidence grew and the experience of being at one with myself completely convinced me that I had found my true calling. How would I become this new Doria – the yoga teacher?

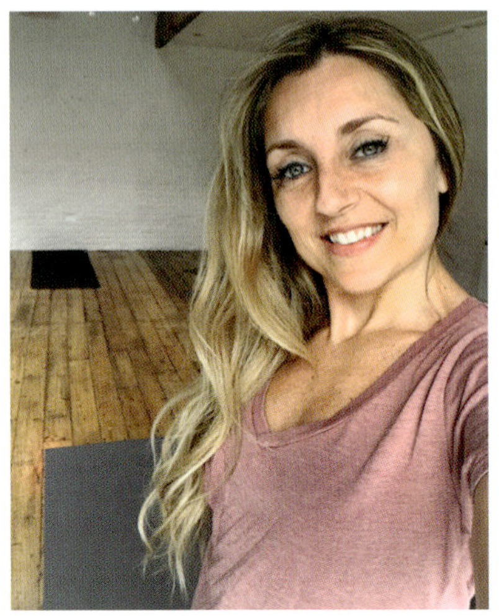

The yoga studio offered me weekly permanent classes straight away, so within a few days I began teaching part-time in a beautiful studio situated just a few minutes from the London Eye.

Teaching was fun and week after week I grew to know the people who were regularly coming to my classes. It was a fulfilling feeling, and I always looked forward to teaching another class. I may have been working two jobs at the time, but I was happy to have found my vocation.

CHAPTER 7

Teaching Yoga

"The best gift you are ever going to give someone— the permission to feel safe in their own skin. To feel worthy. To feel like they are enough."
– Hannah Brencher

Teaching yoga gave me the opportunity to grow as a person and as a teacher. It kept me balanced and focused. It took me beyond the physical practice, on a path of spiritual awakening. There is an intimacy that happens when we decide to share space with people who are willing to put their heart and soul into the beautiful practice of yoga. It's an honour and a privilege and I am thankful for that.

Being at the front of a class and leading a room of people can be intimidating. To this day, I take my seat on my mat at the front of the room and take a deep breath before I start talking, because people are taking time out of their day to listen to what I have to say and guide them on their yoga journey. It's gratifying and at the same time scary. How can my words affect them? Will they be perceived the way I want them to?

I would like to make a difference and I believe that starts with reaching out to others. I love knowing that I'm helping to enhance the lives of the students who come to my classes. Being able to provide a break from the stress of their jobs, family, and the chattering voices in their minds is invigorating. Providing a safe space for people to let go and deeply connect with their body is priceless. Hearing people say how relaxed they are after my class and how they notice a difference if they can't make it to a class is truly gratifying.

I think I'm not only holding space for them, but I believe that I am also teaching them how to hold space for themselves. It's important to me to get to know the people who attend my classes. Knowing their names and who they are as well as what brings them to their mats is essential in being able to connect to their practice and keep them interested in growing.

One of my goals is to create a community that offers a safe space to pursue this growth. Sharing a flow of positive energy that can be passed on, one person at a time, one moment at a time, is an experience that I am truly grateful for. Yoga is a lifelong journey. I am both a student and a teacher at the same time. I will never stop learning.

I believe that all students come to my classes for a reason. Whatever the reason is, it can be a learning experience for the student or a learning experience for me, or both. It may be that the student comes once and never comes back or it may be that someone is ripe to receive what I have to offer, and we develop a long teacher/student relationship over time.

I've stopped trying to decide if meaningful coincidence is true and real or not. I have decided there's some reason why every student walks into my teaching space. Maybe they want to get stronger and become more flexible, maybe they are dealing with a loss of identity, or facing illness for the first time, battling body shame or recovering from an injury. All paths are welcome, as long as they respect each other.

One of my successes has been teaching yoga to people affected by eating disorders. These people have a strong dislike of their bodies and usually want to become smaller and invisible. The first change that has to happen is a desire to have a good relationship with your own body. From there you can move to giving your body the fuel it needs to give you energy. After accepting that food is a good thing for your body's health, you can introduce the idea of getting stronger through eating a healthy diet and regular exercise. Progressing through these stages takes a long time.

I'm not a doctor but by teaching yoga one-to-one and developing a personal relationship with a client, sometimes offering additional coaching sessions, I could see that the effect of the yoga was helping them to heal. I had to make it clear from the outset that it was their responsibility to take care of their own body. It was not my job to cure them or make them happy. My job was to give them the skills to practise yoga and to encourage self-care so that they could heal themselves.

One young woman disliked drinking water. I had to tell her that we weren't going to do any yoga unless she drank some water at the start of every class as her body could not function properly without water. Drinking water for her was as difficult as swallowing a thick protein shake, but she persevered and slowly she began to connect with the needs of her own body and to understand them. Practising yoga requires you to get in touch with your body-mind and in this way, the young woman began to connect on a deeper level and to gradually ignore her anxiety about her body image.

When you see your students making significant progress, it brings a good deal of pride and satisfaction as their teacher.

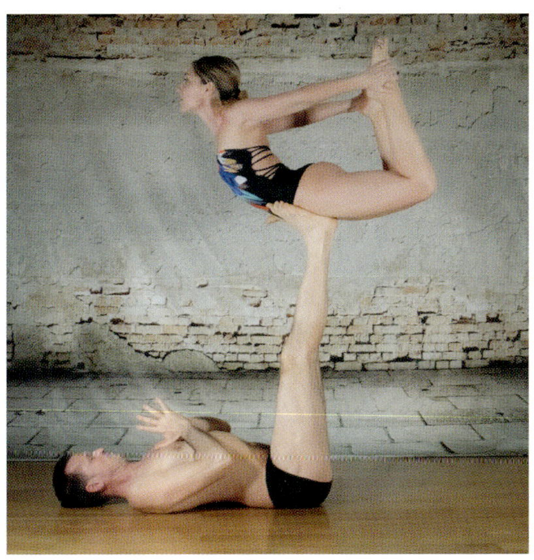

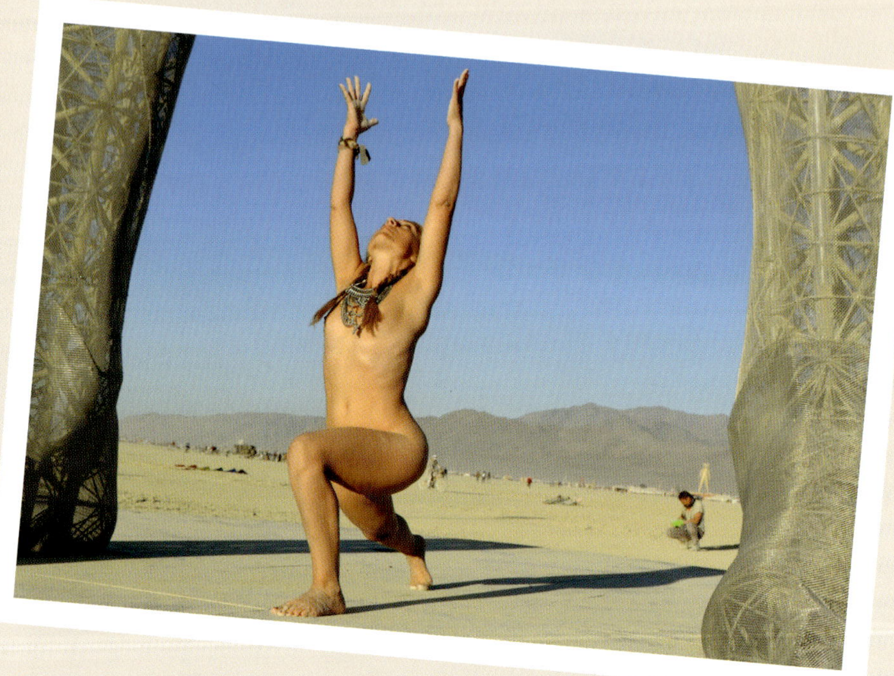

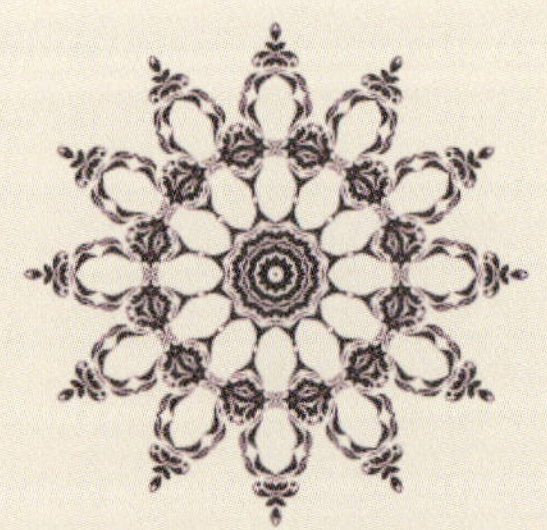

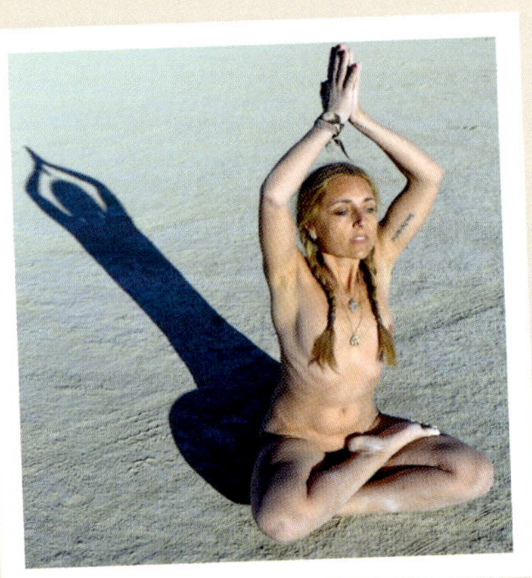

CHAPTER 8

Yoga In The Desert

"When you discover your self-worth, you will lose interest in anyone who doesn't see it."
– Doe Zantamata

In 2015, a friend of mine invited me to the Burning Man Festival. Burning Man is not a typical festival as no acts are booked to perform there, but rather it's the coming together of a global community of people who share the same ethos. I'd heard great things about it and wanted to experience it for myself.

There are ten guiding principles associated with the Burning Man community which they promote on their website (www.burningman.org). They are a blueprint for a holistic way of living that I admire and would encourage others to try, so I include them here:

Radical Inclusion

Gifting

Decommodification

Radical Self-reliance

Radical Self-expression

Communal Effort

Civic Responsibility

Leaving No Trace

Participation

Immediacy

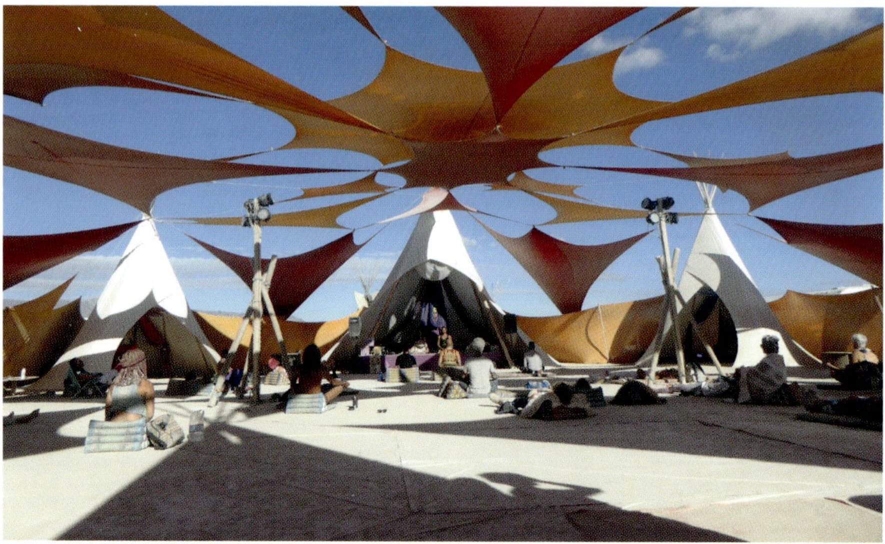

Burning Man now has a global network of thousands of 'Burners' who stage events internationally but it began over thirty years ago in 1986 on a beach in San Francisco when co-founders Larry Harvey and Jerry James first built an effigy of a man and set it on fire with a handful of onlookers as a kind of protest against the rules and strictures of the modern world.

Now it's hard to get hold of one of the 70,000 tickets to the week-long event which some describe as a 24/7 party, and others regard as a beacon of hope for humanity to come together, get creative and discuss utopian ideas. Landscape art is at the centre of each festival with grants given to artists for a range of extraordinary sculptures and art installations that are erected for the duration, some of which are burned at the end. In the evenings, the festival transforms into a magical kind of amusement park where you can dance, sing, wrestle or play with fire.

During the week a temporary structure known as the 'temple' is constructed and solemnly set on fire so that spiritual cleansing can occur by enabling a symbolic farewell to loss and grief. At the end of the week on the Saturday, there is the ritual burning of a 40ft high wooden figure known as the Man. Since this is considered to be Burning Man's equivalent to New Year's Eve, there are fireworks and a collective celebration to mark the event.

*

For me, the trip to Nevada was a life-changing experience. While at the festival, I saw people working collectively for the first time, to make all sorts of things, have fun, share art, or perform dance and drama. What was radical was that it was created in the spirit of people giving something to each other without expectation of any kind of payment or return. Money was only usable to buy bags of ice and/or coffee. The energy of the place was contagious. It was a complete contrast to Reno or Las Vegas where you see people addicted to the endless rows of slot machines in casinos open day and night.

The setting for Burning Man is in the vast alkali flats of the Black Rock desert, with the arid Jackson Mountains and the Calico Hills all around as a backdrop. People arrive in vehicles of all kinds, wearing whatever they wish, some sporting elaborate costumes while others just cover themselves in a layer of sand. They pitch tents or sleep in camper vans and wander around to find out what's going on.

My friends and I stayed in a minivan for seven nights, without a shower. Fruit, protein bars and drinking water were all we had to survive. We brought bicycles, sleeping bags and warm outdoor blankets, an inflatable mattress, emergency kit, baby wipes and lots of water. There were camps set up all over the Playa, (which is how the site is described), offering all manner of free things from vodka to massage to bicycle repair to hot steaming food.

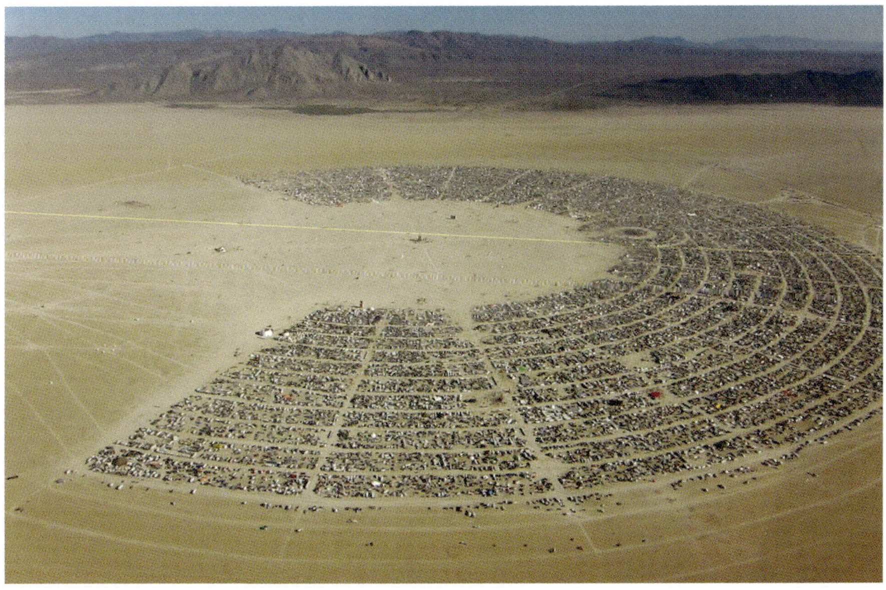

Aerial view of the Burning Man Festival Grounds in 2010. Photo Kyle Harmon

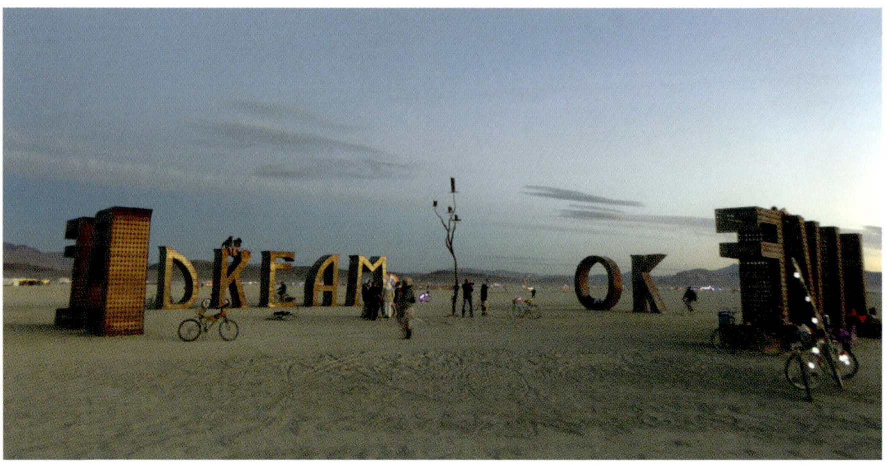

One morning I woke up very early, got on my bike and started to explore this extraordinary place in the middle of nowhere. Not many people were around that early, but there was art everywhere I looked, beautiful colours, and the gentle sound of music of every kind.

One of the art installations comprised giant-sized letters spelling the words BE, DREAM, OK and LIVE. As you wander around you experience a sense of awe at the absurdity and bizarre nature of it all. The aim is to inspire you to downshift from a consumer lifestyle, and to participate by giving freely to other people.

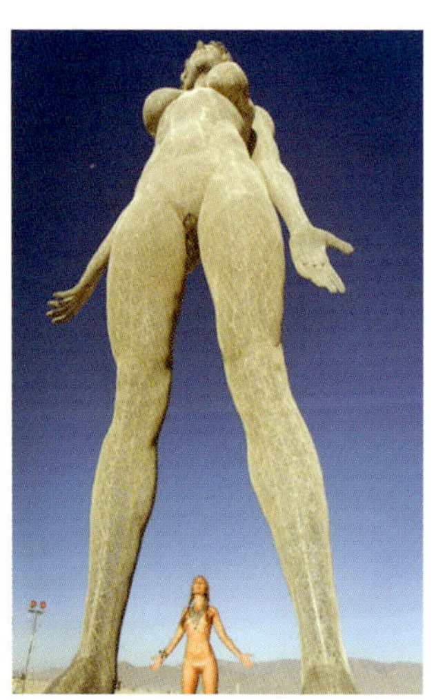

R-evolution by Marco Cochrane

Nudity is one of the ways people divest themselves of the usual social conventions and decorating yourself with body paint is a popular choice. However, seasoned 'Burners' have learned to sport sturdy footwear, take goggles to protect their eyes from the regular dust storms and to wear some kind of head gear to avoid heat stroke in the baking hot terrain.

As I was cycling around I noticed a huge art installation which was about 45ft high, depicting a woman in a standing yoga position called 'Mountain Pose'.[1] This giant sculpture was not only incredible to look at, but she had an air compressor installed in her chest, which meant

---

1. http://www.marcocochranesculpture.net/r-evolution

that she seemed to be breathing! It was fascinating, and I stopped to take some pictures.

At that moment, a woman nearby took her clothes off and posed in front of the sculpture for a photo shoot. She had beautiful, blonde curly hair, and I guessed she was a professional model, the way she posed so naturally, although she was completely naked. I felt envious, imagining that it would have been thrilling to do something like that. But then I told myself it was a crazy idea, jumping completely out of my comfort zone like that. I'd regret it later, wouldn't I? But I also thought perhaps I'd regret *not* doing it later? It was like I had a devil and an angel sitting on my shoulders pulling me this way and that. Yes, no, yes, no, until I burst out: "I'm gonna f***ing do this!"

The photo shoot was soon over. Without a second thought I approached another professional photographer to ask if he would take some photographs of me. I made it clear that I wanted some photos of myself performing naked yoga, to prove that I had actually done it, when I was back in Britain. "Yes, of course," he replied.

The purple streaks of the dawn were spreading beyond the darkness of the mountains. It was a beautiful experience. I could feel the sun warming my skin as I performed the movements with my eyes closed, focusing on my breathing. As I got into the flow of the yoga, I felt as if I were being cleansed of my shame and fear.

When I opened my eyes, a crowd had gathered around me. They were not laughing or mocking me but watching appreciatively and applauding; some were calling out, "Cool!" and "You go, girl!" That made me smile.

It was in the Black Rock desert that I found true freedom. I faced my twin demons there: fear and shame. I learned that being naked can set you free and I went away from Burning Man with a mission – to help others to find that sense of liberation too.

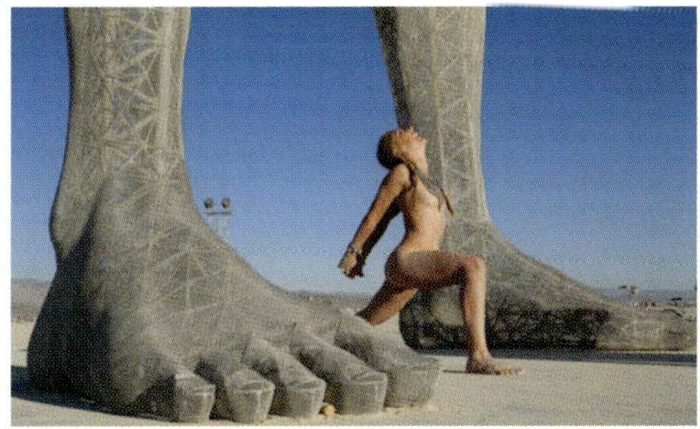

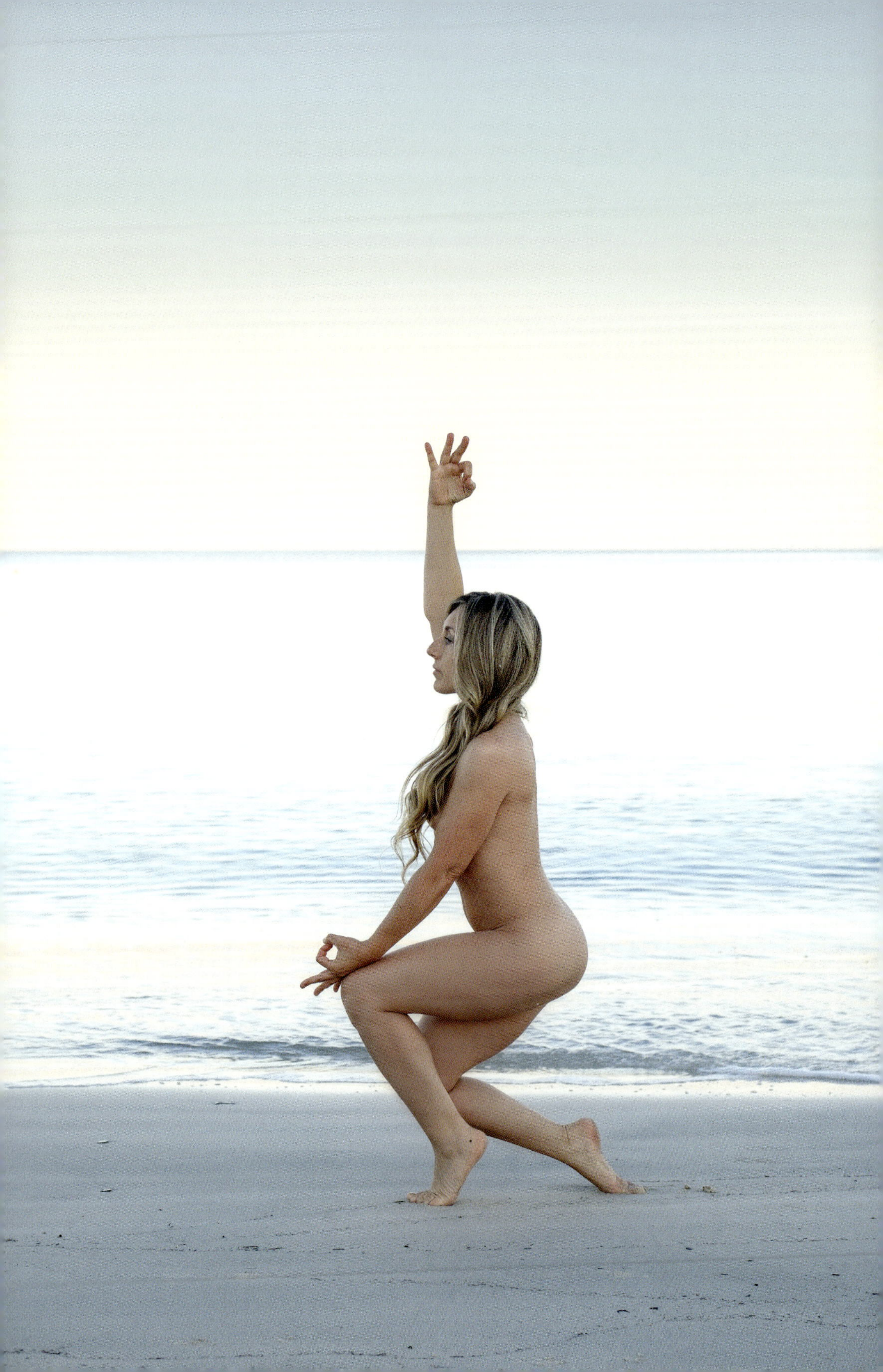

CHAPTER 9

Becoming A Naked Yoga Teacher

"The most revolutionary thing you can do is love your body."
(Unknown)

Back in the UK, the idea of teaching naked yoga seemed laughable. Only a few people were doing it and there didn't seem to be any demand. To be honest, I was concerned about what others would say or how I might be judged if I started to offer naked yoga classes. But my experience at Burning Man had planted the idea in my mind and it wouldn't go away.

A few weeks later, I was signing up on one of the international yoga teaching websites: name, surname, address and what kind of yoga style do you teach. Many boxes to be ticked, Vinyasa, ticked, power yoga, ticked, yin yoga, ticked, restorative yoga, ticked, meditation, ticked, naked yoga… and there it was, this naked yoga shadow was following me again. I took a deep breath, and I ticked that box too.

The next morning as I opened my email, I noticed an incredible number of notifications from that website. I was overwhelmed by messages from people asking for information about the naked yoga classes. I suddenly understood why I'd had this premonition: I was going to become a naked yoga teacher.

It wasn't plain sailing to go ahead with the classes despite the obvious need. My inner critic was in overdrive in the days before I started. There were a few others teaching naked yoga around the world and I tried to learn as much as I could from studying their websites. I signed up for a class myself with another naked yoga practitioner to see how they conducted the class and was impressed with the natural way in which our collective nudity was treated in a small space. It gave me the courage I needed to go ahead.

But there were no obvious role models to follow and, in the end, I had to work out the rules for the classes by myself. I was frightened of what might happen and how I would handle it. But every pioneer has to take a step into the unknown, and so it was with me. My career as a naked yoga teacher was launched in a chilly community hall in south London in April 2016, and I haven't looked back.

One of the things I have learned as a naked yoga teacher is that it is important to evaluate new students – and to understand their intentions. Those who are genuine about joining a class often express their anxieties about practising naked yoga straight away. Students tend to share their struggles with me about their body image and the fact that they cannot overcome their negative thoughts about certain aspects of their body.

One-to-One Classes

When teaching one-to-one classes, students often come to my studio first, where I ask them to fill out a form with their details, discover if they have any injuries or have had any recent operations and learn more about them as people. For example, I like to know about their diet and lifestyle, if they eat organic food, are vegetarian, meat-eaters or drink alcohol. Also, it's important to discuss whether they consume enough water each day and if they have a regular exercise routine.

It's also important to know if they sit at a desk in their work or if they are active and do a physical job like being a builder or a waitress, or if they work with kids or as carers which can be demanding emotionally.

Then I ask about their perception of their body, their previous experiences, their family's attitudes and if they are satisfied with their life in general. I like to understand what brought them there, and why they want to practise naked yoga.

Some of my students want to reconnect with their bodies, some want to love themselves again, some want to learn how to relax after a long day at work, and others want to find a way to fight all the negative thoughts that they have about themselves. This sometimes leads on to life coaching sessions in cases where specific issues have been raised which the student and I agree require deeper and further discussion.

During the one-to-one session, I explain our aims for the class, based on the program I have designed for that particular student's needs. I begin by teaching all my students the correct way to breathe during a yoga class and the connection between the breath and the body. I teach them the basis of meditation so they can practise at home and when travelling.

Depending on the reasons for wanting to practise naked yoga, I design the class to deliver the student's desired outcomes, for example we will do a more relaxing session if the student is there because of stress or we will undertake a stronger practice if they like to sweat or if they prefer more physically challenging exercises.

I always ask for feedback during the class, especially if a certain position doesn't feel comfortable, and then I offer modifications. At the end of the class we finish with *Shavasana* (final relaxation) where the student lays down completely relaxed on the floor for about five minutes. Then we sit up in a crossed-legged position on the mat and we close the session.

Some men worry about getting an erection when they first come to a naked yoga class. They ask questions like: "How will I cope?" "Will people laugh at me?" Yoga moves a lot of energy around the body. Erections are not limited to sexual attraction and can occur quite spontaneously. If you find that you have an erection, simply carry on with the movements. It is likely to subside after a few minutes because of the physical nature of Vinyasa yoga. There is certainly no need to feel embarrassed.

Group Classes

For the group class I like to burn some incense to prepare the room and create a more spiritual atmosphere. I keep the lights soft, ensure that it's warm by using infrared lamps, and play relaxing music like 'Buddha Bar'.

The studio is completely private and the yoga mats are arranged in a horseshoe or circular pattern around the teacher so that each person faces the teacher but is not looking directly at anyone else – and nobody is behind another person. I do understand that we are all sexual beings but the class is not the place for sexual energy nor the place for making a sexual connection. I'm very strict in providing a safe space which is not for sexual nudity.

I have devised a set of rules for the in-person group classes:

- Students must be over 18 years of age to attend any mixed-gender class.
- Photography, physical contact and staring at another student are strictly prohibited.
- Students can bring their own mats or use the mats that are provided at the studio.
- If they borrow a mat from the studio they have to bring a towel to place on top of the mat for hygiene and protection.
- Nudity is mandatory so everybody will be on the same level. Women are allowed to wear pants or shorts during their menstrual cycle.
- Only positive vibes in the class; no criticism of others.
- Any misconduct will result in being excluded from the class and from any future bookings without a refund.

Online Classes

In addition to the rules above we maintain the following:

- Each session is hosted online and requires the participant to have their camera on, be in view, and to be participating. Unfortunately, if these conditions cannot be met, even for technical reasons, the student will be removed from the session.
- Students are free to play their own music during the class or they can play the Spotify playlist that I send with the zoom link.
- I mute the students' microphones before we start the practice.
- When I start teaching I don't face the screen, students see me on the side so they can properly see the movements of the yoga sequences.
- At the end of the class students can give me feedback, raise questions or talk to each other.

Over the years, I have had the privilege to teach people from all walks of life and of all ages, some of whom found that naked yoga enhanced the joy they felt in being alive, or it gave them the strength to change their lives.

*

Here's an extract from my blog written after I'd been teaching naked yoga classes for a year:

Exactly 12 months ago I taught my first co-ed naked yoga class in London.

I remember I was so scared of being judged that even the idea of it made me feel sick.

Despite the fact that I was petrified of teaching in a room full of naked strangers, I put my 'super confident naked yoga teacher' mask on, and I taught the first of many naked yoga classes.

Looking back today, I feel proud of myself for always fighting my fears. I feel grateful for all the beautiful people who crossed my naked yoga path, and I feel blessed for every person I had the privilege to help to overcome their body issues.

I'm providing a safe place where people can truly and deeply be themselves; they can experience the powerful confidence that comes with practising naked.

Naked yoga is not sex and if you still relate a naked body with sexuality you are not ready for this – and probably you never will be.

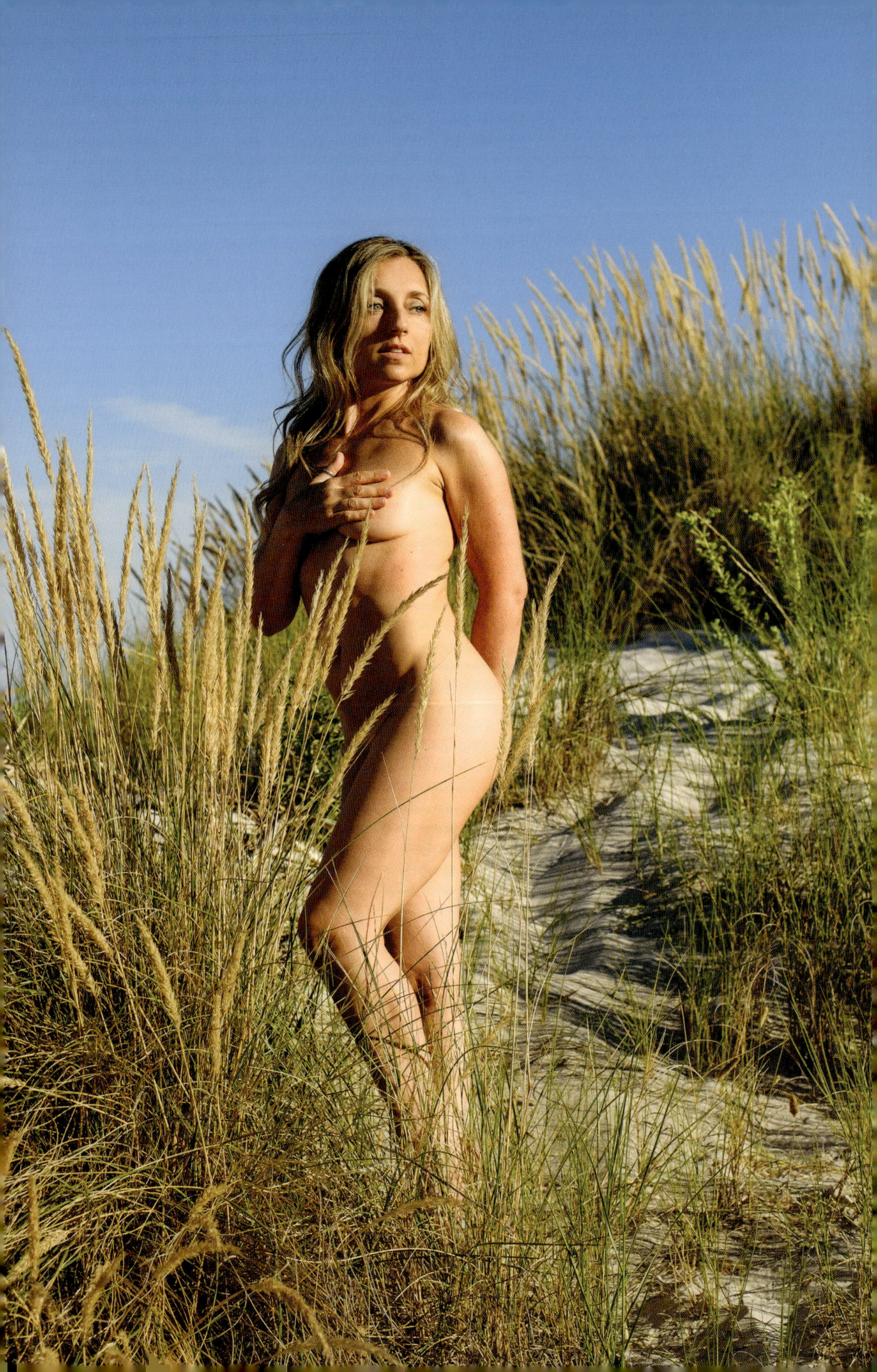

CHAPTER 10

Fighting Body Shame With Naked Yoga

"Shame derives its power from being unspeakable."
– Brene Brown

One year later of teaching one-to-one classes, my work as a naked yoga teacher expanded beyond offering group classes to adults. I now also teach couples and one-to-one sessions for those who have special needs. Some of my students are suffering from depression, eating disorders, gender identity disorders (GIDs) and various conditions all leading to body shame.

From witnessing the positive benefits that people have received from practising naked yoga in my classes, I truly consider naked yoga as a powerful tool to demystify body shame and to empower people to accept their own body, embracing all their imperfections. I feel proud of the work I have done and that I am doing because it is making a positive difference to people's lives.

After my operation and the period of disorientation that followed, I decided that I didn't want to live my old life anymore, but I didn't know how to go about creating a new life. For things to change I learned that you need to take risks, try out new things, set new goals and go for them. I was sick, lost, broke, fearful and ashamed back in those days. Now I have new self-respect and I am no longer holding myself back from pursuing the things I want to do.

One of the things I decided that I wanted, was to have a healthy, lean and muscular body. To achieve this, I worked with a professional nutritionist along with training twice a day to get really fit. The key is to set intentions with determination and not give up.

Although I love drinking good champagne, eating good food and having a good time, I have realised that to live a physically and mentally healthy life, these things need to be in moderation.

I also have a daily skin care routine. This is not vanity but a way of showing that you care for your body every day, in the morning and the evening. I use natural oils like CBD, and these give me both pleasure and the skin tone I want to have – especially given I am naked much of my day teaching naked yoga.

As part of my work, I also offer to coach people to achieve a better life. One of the things that always surprises me is that most people would rather stay doing what they do for a living, even though they often don't feel fulfilled, than make the effort to change. In many cases they find it easier to take their clothes off in public than reach out for the life they really want. I see my job as helping them have the courage to do both, hopefully becoming both happy and fit along the way.

The biggest challenge for a lot of people is to allow self-loving to happen. Once we start being kinder to ourselves and we stop putting up barriers as to why we shouldn't do it or why we don't deserve it, the relief and feeling of warmth and comfort is immense.

Moreover, once I learned to love myself, I found that I could go deeper with this love, and, like all love, this has helped me to stay mentally and physically fit for the many years that I have been cancer-free.

Challenging your inner critic and not paying any heed to the negative dialogue going on inside your head is another path to a mentally healthy life. For some of us, this negative voice is louder than for others, but we all have it. I now know that meditation and moments of stillness along with self-love are a critical part of my armoury to stay mentally healthy and to be able to teach my clients from a place of calm. I meditate every day so that I can help my clients get to a place of peace and quiet too. Having a calm internal world enables them to get more connected to their bodies and get more benefit from their naked yoga practice each day.

The freedom you feel from being naked also gives you the courage to be yourself in all aspects of your life, be it work, family, sexuality or spirituality.

I have a tattoo on my arm that sums up how I feel about life and it says:

"My Life My Way"

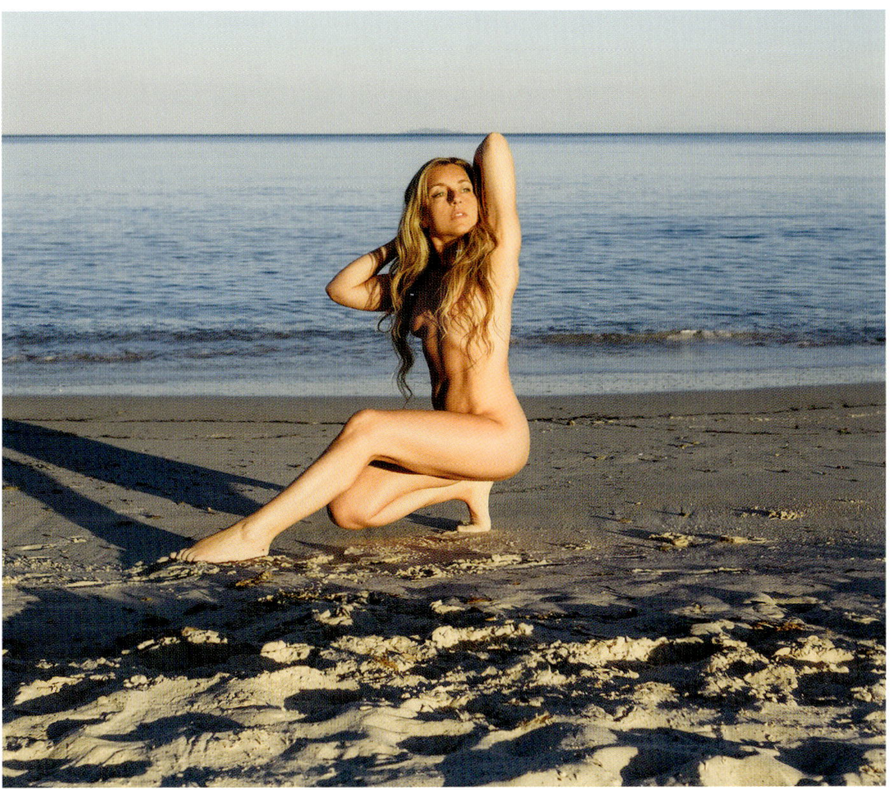

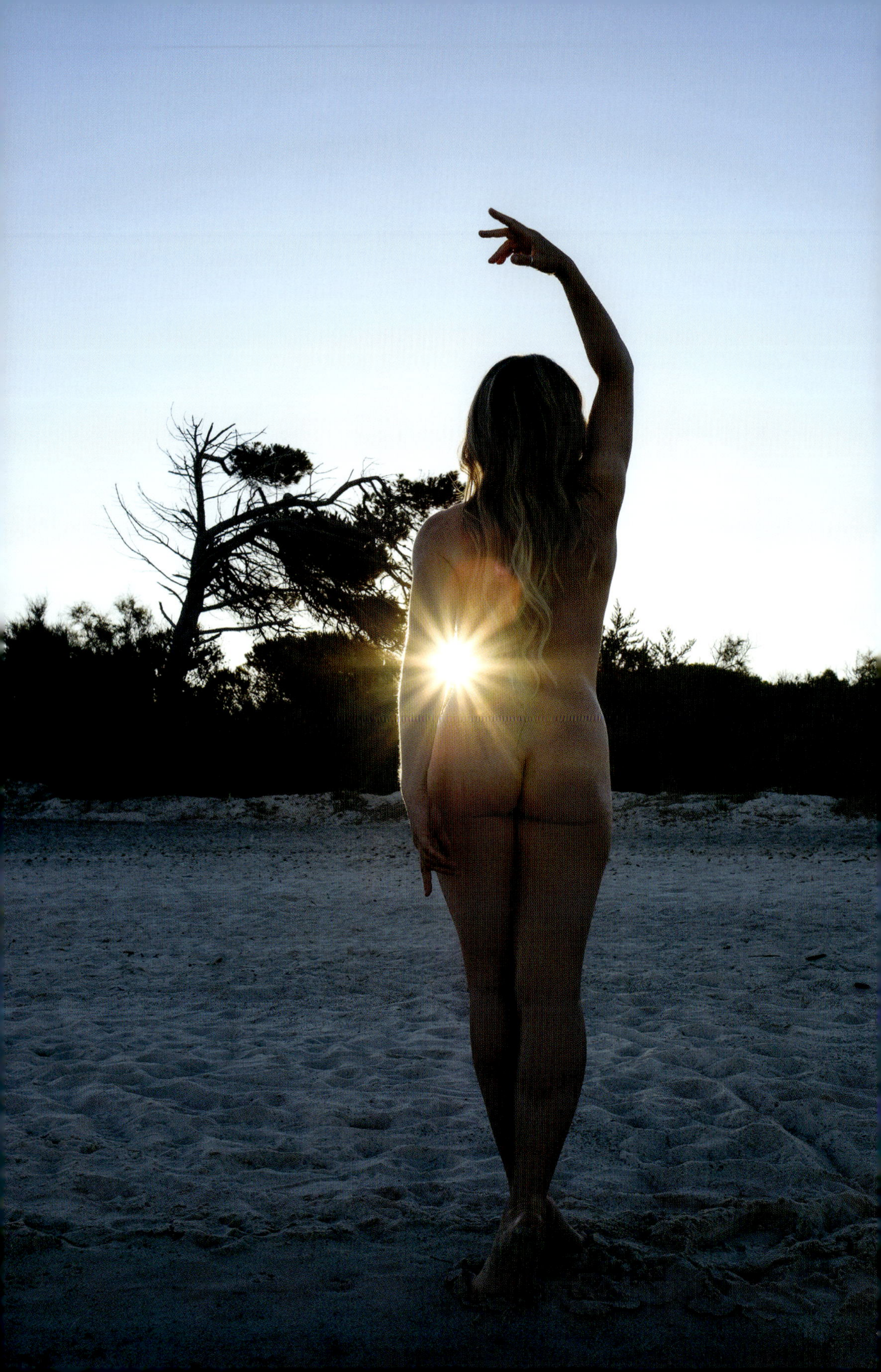

CHAPTER 11

Taking Naked Yoga Online

The lockdowns due to Covid-19 brought a lot of change for most of us. We had to stay inside, or it was at least recommended, depending on where you were.

The first lockdown pushed many to their limit. Whether you were by yourself and cut off from your usual social contacts or forced to spend all your time with your family/roommates, many had to adapt to a new reality. Both scenarios put a lot of pressure on individuals. On top of this, many lost their jobs or had to be creative and courageous and adapt like me.

People were frightened during the first lockdown in the UK, but due to government mixed messaging, there were many who felt annoyed when the second lockdown was introduced in November 2020. Some questioned why the situation was different in the autumn, when it had been possible to meet up outside and spend your free time outdoors in the summer.

Not being able to see your loved ones or do the things you usually do to relax and enjoy yourself (like attending that Monday evening yoga class), brought challenges for many people's mental health and left many crying out for relief.

I could see that people needed to develop a healthy exercise regime and good self-care while stuck indoors. It was a new challenge to deal with the technology and marketing necessary to set up and offer online yoga classes, but I quickly was able to provide a range of options to my students for them to join with others in a safe, communal online environment.

The combination of movement, meditation and breath-work, together with being live online with people from all over the world, helped to ground people and enabled them to connect with themselves and others. Some were even inspired to create their own little yoga corner at home, a space reserved for unwinding and relaxation, dedicated to time spent on the mat.

Before Covid-19, I'd had the idea of teaching online but kept postponing putting it into action. I felt anxious about doing it because I didn't feel like I was good enough to put myself out there nor that I was ready to handle any negativity. On top of this, there was a rush by my yoga and fitness colleagues to take their classes online too, to make up for lost in-studio sessions, meaning there was a lot of competition.

I wasn't sure where to begin, but after some research, I took a few hesitant steps to offer my naked yoga online and started my online teaching journey. It was nerve-wracking at first to get in front of the camera, but eventually, I managed to get over my fears. Now I am grateful I did and wouldn't want it any other way. It is not only keeping me connected with my community of students, affectionately called 'Doritos', but also keeping me sane, happy and grounded. Teaching online has brought me even closer to my community.

The anxiety and fear I had around teaching on-screen are now gone. More importantly, I'm glad I have been able to keep teaching during this difficult time and have found it to be working well for me and my lifestyle. I am planning on continuing to offer online 'live' classes even after the Covid-19 crisis, as it has opened up new opportunities to teach people from all over the world on a regular basis, instead of exclusively Londoners.

On a technical level, I have had positive experiences using Zoom. I can see my students, and they can see each other if they wish. My students report that it feels like being in the room together – connecting, moving, breathing and practising with other yogis at the same time.

In advance of my classes, I prepare playlists which I send out for students to play during the class if they wish. I put all of my students on mute during the session to ensure good sound quality. This way they can only hear my voice and not everybody else's background noise.

At the beginning of the first lockdown, I felt slightly lost, not entirely sure how to proceed and how to have a continuous income to pay my bills. Teaching online has given me back my sense of purpose and direction. It fills me with joy and happiness to receive messages from my students all over the world, telling me how good they feel after a class and how happy they are that we can practise together, especially during difficult times when we need to connect more than ever.

In this pandemic, when so many have lost loved ones, people have opened their hearts and shown compassion towards each other through channels like social media, Zoom, etc. Previously, people were using social media to promote a perfect picture of their lives, but in this time of crisis, social media provided an opportunity to receive sympathy, advice, practical help and humour in the face of a natural calamity. The lockdowns have led to a re-evaluation of what we really care about, making people more honest and authentic in what they are sharing of themselves online.

Even though the circumstances are distressing, this is an opportunity for us to learn the difference between reaction and response. We can reassess what is truly important and worthy of our energy. Furthermore, it allows us time to see what we already have, not just what we've lost. In order to understand what self-love is, we need to feel the proverbial ground beneath our feet. We have a chance to explore how we can put our years of practice into play and look beyond the self. It also challenges us to get creative with how we stay united and support and hold space for each other.

This global pandemic has been a huge wake-up call, and people are recognising the value of staying healthy and reducing stress which is harmful to the immune system. The world needs yoga, now more than ever. Yoga can provide a refuge, a chance to breathe and recover from the stresses of daily life, but it also allows you to cultivate the tools and resources to be in a graceful relationship with all that arises, come what may.

During lockdown, many people were trying to create some sort of routine for themselves to avoid feeling lost and alone. Many of them re-discovered yoga during the lockdown and noticed a vast improvement in their ability to stay calm or maintain mental stability. Keeping mentally and physically well became a new priority. The benefits of yoga for the mind as well as the body are well documented, and it's clear that regular practice aids wellbeing. I'm honoured that people from all around the world made space in their lives to practise their yoga with me.

As humans we are social creatures, depending on human connection and social interaction. We need to have close and healthy relationships in order to live a happy and fulfilled life. Harvard University started their ongoing study into predictors of old age in 1939. Today, the original participants' children and grandchildren are taking part in the study and answering questions about their life on a regular basis. Obviously, taking care of yourself by avoiding smoking and drinking alcohol, eating a healthy diet and staying fit, all contribute to a person's chances of living into old age. Not surprisingly, factors that shorten the lifespan are poverty and poor education. But the number one factor to ensure a person ages well is having stable and close relationships with others. Being part of a community matters.

Even though I was hesitant in the beginning about teaching online and wondering if it would be possible to create a good and relaxing atmosphere, I have found that an intimate and welcoming setting is possible. When teaching naked yoga, creating the right atmosphere is key. For newer people, I offer the chance to enter the online room first to have a chat about how they feel about nudity. Later on, everyone has to have their camera turned on in order to create a safe space.

By offering online live yoga classes, I combine physical exercise (as well as meditation and breath-work) and human connection. For my regular in-person students who have been practising together for some time and who know each other, it provides a chance to see each other and to reconnect. For newer clients, it gives them a chance to meet new people and make new connections.

One thing I have encountered many times while promoting body positivity and teaching naked yoga online is people relating nudity to sex. Educating people about the difference between the two is one of my life goals. One of the downsides of being online is dealing with those who post negative comments. People hide behind their (anonymous) online profile, which gives them a sense of safety and makes it easy for them to attack and criticise others.

We are all born naked. Nudity is our natural state of being. Being naked is being in your truest form; it reveals your essence. When we are naked, we are vulnerable. Vulnerability does not equal sexualisation at all, as it takes courage to show yourself as you truly are. Becoming comfortable in your own skin is a great advantage in life for both men and women, but especially for women whose bodies are objectified and sexualized in the arts and media on a daily basis.

Many of my students are nervous when they first attend one of my online classes and they feel shy and hesitant when entering the online room. As soon as they realise that there is no sexual energy directed at them or anyone else, and it is all about yoga, they relax. Seeing others being comfortable in their own skin gives them permission to feel the same way and over time they build greater confidence in themselves as human beings.

Let us be great role models and teach our kids that nudity is the norm and nothing to hide or be ashamed of. It is time to connect on a primal level as naked human beings, irrespective of body size, disability, race, class or sexuality.

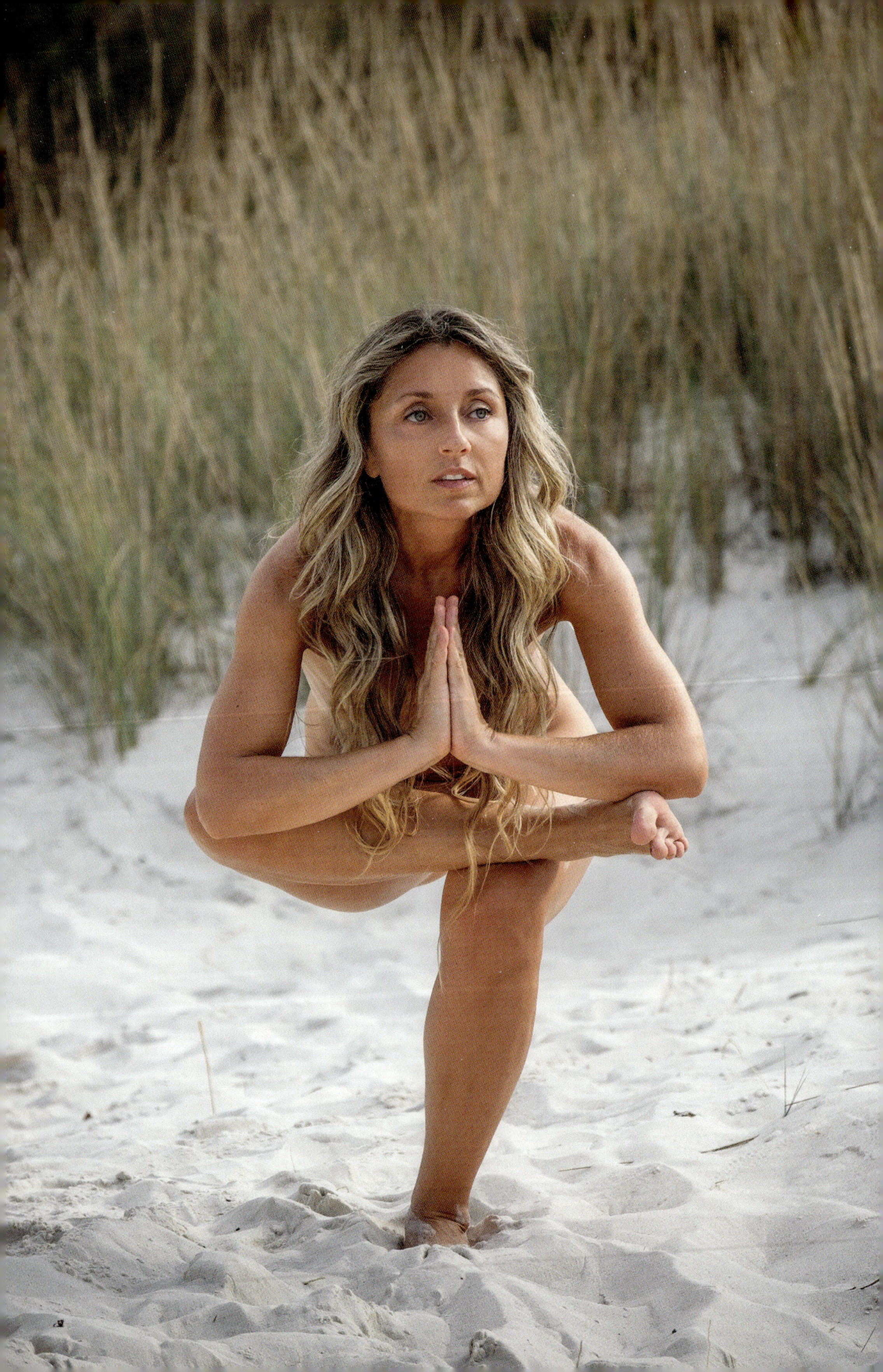

PART TWO

Connect With Your Body

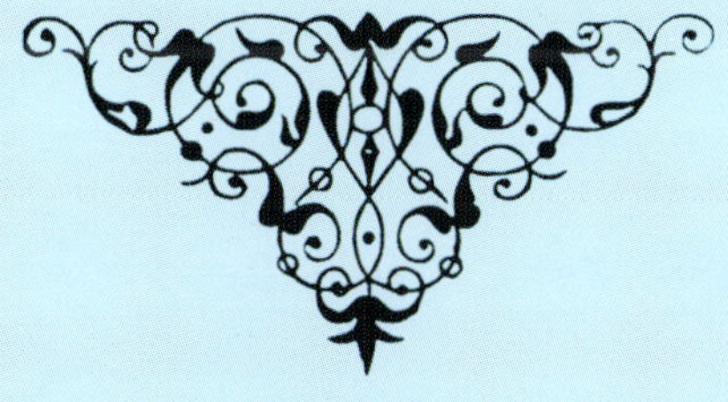

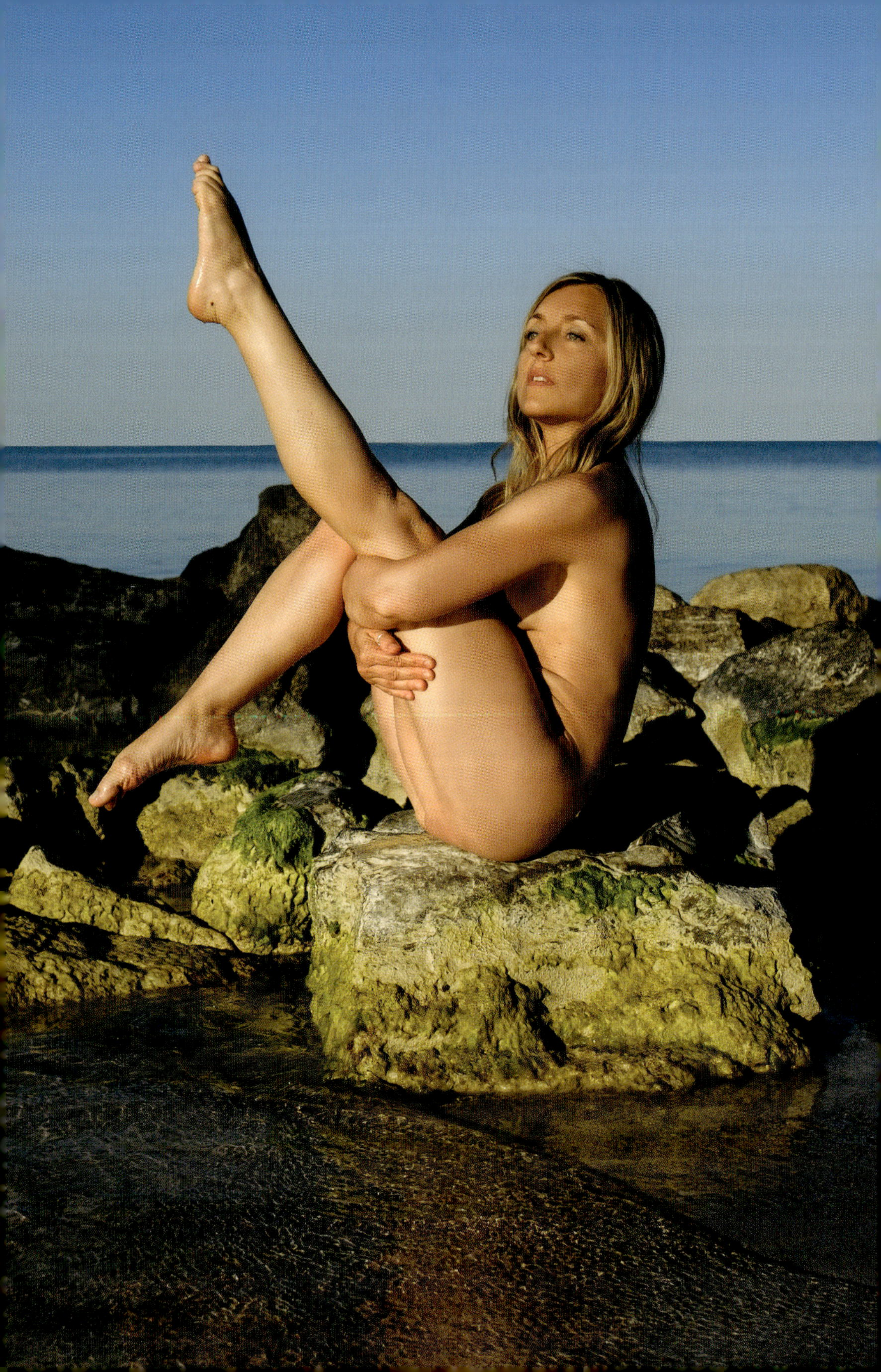

CHAPTER 12

How To Get Confident Naked

*"Confidence will make you happier than any diet ever will.
So, embrace your body."*
(Unknown)

Below you will find a list of things and activities you can do to increase your confidence being naked:

Practise naked yoga:

Practising yoga naked normalises being naked – by yourself and around others. By stripping down the outer facade that is clothed in a secure space, you learn that it is safe to be naked and vulnerable. You stop judging others, and instead, start to appreciate yourself and others more. It also increases your self-confidence, as you are challenged to step out of your comfort zone. On a more practical level, you don't have to tuck in your shirt after every sun salute, and there are no itchy yoga pants.

Don't compare yourself to presumed perfection (perfection doesn't even exist):

In Western society, we are chasing literally made-up beauty standards, that a natural human being cannot achieve without surgery etc. No face is completely symmetrical, and yet we have it in our minds that this is what we need to look like. Next time you see an advert or a perfect picture of someone, remind yourself of the fact that this is not real, and ask yourself who is profiting from you feeling bad about yourself (like beauty and dieting companies, for example). Then, put down that magazine.

Practise naked gardening:

If you have a private garden, which is closed off to the neighbours, make use of this privilege and do some naked gardening. Feeling the earth between your toes and your fingers will connect you deeply with mother earth and ground you immediately. These sensory feelings send a response to your brain to calm you and slow down your breathing.

Practise naked hiking:

Walking barefoot stimulates the muscles in your feet more, and improves balance and the mechanics of hips, knees and core. Combining this with the freedom nudity brings, it's the perfect recipe for an unforgettable experience. There are also naked hiking clubs where you can learn to accept and be accepted by others. In Europe, due to demand, there are special trails devoted to hiking nude. Please be aware that nudity can be illegal and may lead to repercussions (such as charges for 'public indecency'), so do your research and look for these special naked hiking trails, and check the popularity of the area you want to walk in.

Practise naked sunbathing:

The more skin is exposed to the sun, the more vitamin D your body produces. This means that naked sunbathing will give you an even tan and may also improve your mood. Whether you sunbathe naked at home by yourself or go to a nudist beach and share the experience with others, relaxing naked will improve your overall wellbeing and help you connect with your body.

Go to a naturist beach:

Seeing others feeling at home in their own bodies will make you feel at ease when going to a naturist beach, and eventually, you will regard human bodies as what they truly are – containers that carry us, beautiful all in their own unique way. Maybe bring along your best friend or your partner and make an adventure of it. There are many websites that provide information on the best nudist beaches around. I even wrote a blogpost about this subject, check it out on my website: www.doriayoga.com

Go to a naturist sauna:

Depending on where you live, and your cultural background, it might be normal to go to a naturist sauna or not. It is actually more hygienic to go naked in a sauna than wearing a swimsuit which encourages the growth of bacteria. Please ensure you always sit on a towel (you can also wrap it around yourself if you feel more comfortable doing so). Bear in mind that there are mixed saunas and others separated by sex (I recommend doing some research first to find what suits you best). Also, make sure it is a safe place for naturists and not a sex sauna, so check the reviews online before going.

Swim naked:

Floating in the water naked is one of the best and most natural feelings. Next time you go for a swim, where possible, do it naked and feel the water gently stroking your body. With every exhale, you can let go a bit more and surrender yourself to the water. Enjoy the freedom and beauty that comes with it and feel how you are carried by the water (especially when swimming in salt water).

Sleep naked:

Sleeping naked is proven to have many health benefits, including improving your sleep quality. Your body temperature will be lower, which helps you to fall asleep more easily, and sleep more deeply. Also you don't have to deal with itchy or uncomfortable nightwear, meaning your body is more comfortable. If you share a bed with your significant other in the nude, it creates more intimacy between you two (not necessarily in a sexual way, but rather feeling close to the other person). If you are going through menopause, sleeping naked can help alleviate the not-so-fun symptoms of hot flushes.

Tone your body:

Sport is proven to have many health benefits. Exercise releases endorphins (which make you feel happy) and helps you to get a better understanding of your body and connect to it. By working out in the gym or doing weight-lifting, you tone your body and become happier, equalling a boost in body confidence. Try starting with ten minutes every day, instead of 90 minutes once a week, to successfully make a habit out of working out.

Improve your posture, look better:

When we are confident, we carry ourselves with pride. We are aware of our own worth, and we look like it. Think of how someone sad walks through life with slouched shoulders. Do you think this makes them feel better or worse? To boost your confidence, improve your posture: make sure you are grounded and carry your body the best way possible. Yoga can be beneficial for this as well.

Go to a naked festival or naturist event:

Once we remove our packaging (clothing), we are all the same – without a suit, an executive is equal to a cashier. Clothes tell stories about people. If there are no clothes, we cannot put people into boxes, but actually have to spend time and effort to find out more about them. Naked festivals and naturist events provide the perfect playground for making new friends without judgement and are a perfect way to learn more about and experience the naturist lifestyle.

Read books about body positivity movements:

Often looking at something from a different angle helps you to realise certain things. Challenge your own beliefs about body image and beauty standards by reading books about body positivity. As there is so much content out there about this topic, nowadays, there is bound to be something you will be able to relate to on a personal level. Read about body positivity to help heal your relationship with your own body.

Watch films/documentaries about body positivity movements:

As already covered, getting information about a topic can help you to broaden your perspective. A great way to do this, is also by watching films and documentaries. Let yourself be inspired by other peoples' take on body positivity, and/or their personal journey to loving and accepting themselves for who they are.

In 2018, I was featured in a body positivity documentary for the East End Film Festival. The short film, *Bare With Me*, questions our relationship with nudity and why we so quickly relate it to sex, fear and loathing. The documentary discusses how people feel about social nudity and aims to explore how confidence in our own bodies and respect for others, prevents objectification and, in extreme cases, harassment, that plagues society. Challenging doubts and false impressions about nudity, is what I do in every one of my naked yoga classes.

Give your body gratitude by standing naked in front of a mirror:

In our modern world, we focus a lot on images, often through social media. This leads to spending time in front of the mirror, comparing ourselves to these images and ideals and criticising our bodies, instead of being grateful. Next time you are in front of a mirror by yourself, strip off your clothes and admire that glorious body of yours which carries you through life every day. Think of all the amazing things your body does for you, day in day out, and say "thank you" (I really encourage you to say these words out loud).

Send positive thoughts to the parts of your body that you don't like:

Next time you look at yourself in the mirror and stare at the mole which has been bothering you for years or catch yourself criticising your body for the way it looks, close your eyes, take a deep breath and send positive thoughts and love to that body part you dislike. Be grateful for your big nose and how it provides you with a constant flow of breath equalling life energy.

Practise naked meditation:

The goal of meditation is to gain a deeper insight into yourself and who you are. Doing it naked means that you are even more raw, more vulnerable and can access deeper layers more deeply. If you lack confidence in your body, start slowly and just sit with the feeling of discomfort. Let it be there and gradually ease into it. This way you can slowly build up your confidence and create a better relationship with yourself. If you struggle with this, I understand – and you don't need to be ashamed.

Dance naked:

Dancing has a lot of proven health benefits. It releases endorphins and tension and is the perfect way to express yourself. It also increases body confidence by giving you a natural mood boost. It has even evolved into its own type of therapy. Dancing naked will let you experience real freedom and help you to be yourself. If this is new for you, try with the lights off, or put on some good tunes and shake it out.

Get a naked massage:

Your body is a mirror of your emotions, like getting hot when upset or tensing up when afraid. We store emotions in our physical bodies and often hold onto them for a long time. A good massage goes into the deeper tissue and can be beneficial in releasing these tensions. Next time you go for a massage, ask the masseuse if it would be okay to be completely naked to connect even deeper with your body.

Naked journaling:

Taking off your clothes, means stripping down layers and tearing down the different masks you have created in your everyday life. You are not just naked physically, but also emotionally. Coming from this state of true self, it is easier to channel all your emotions (comfortable and uncomfortable ones) and write them into a diary or journal.

Naked pranayama (breathing):

Pranayama promotes relaxation and mindfulness. It also improves lung function, lowers high blood pressure, and increases brain function. Doing pranayama without any constricting yoga pants or other clothes allows you to breathe even deeper and furthermore connect more fully with your body and your breath.

CHAPTER 13

How To Love Yourself

"You can't hate yourself happily. You can't criticise yourself thin. You can't shame yourself wealthy. Real change begins with self-love and self-care."
– Jessica Ortner

Over the past few decades, we have seen a trend of unrealistic beauty ideals. The images we are fed by the media are literally unachievable, photoshopped standards and ideals. Many of us struggle with loving and accepting ourselves and our body. A lot of us define ourselves by our exterior. We base our self-worth on outside validation instead of validating ourselves for who we are as a person and how we show up in the world.

Loving yourself means treating yourself with kindness, using loving words when talking to or about yourself and giving yourself the support needed. As you are the only person you have to spend every second of your life with, make this relationship count by investing in it. Imagine you are talking to your best friend, who you love and adore, and then treat yourself in the same way. Be the person who shows up for yourself, whatever happens. Ensure to listen to your own needs and act accordingly, say "yes" to yourself, even if this means saying "no" to others. One easy thing, you can start doing today is looking at yourself in the mirror naked and telling yourself that you are a beautiful, worthy human being.

Here below, you will find some tips about how to love yourself and embrace your imperfections.

Loving yourself is not an option, it is mandatory:

Who, if not yourself, will love you and always have your best interests at heart? You need to understand that others will treat you the way you treat yourself. If you don't have high standards in this regard, others won't accept your boundaries. By changing your relationship with yourself, you are changing all of your other relationships too. Self-love is a must. With self-compassion and kindness, you can go from self-acceptance to liking and eventually loving yourself. Be gentle with yourself, know that there are ups and downs, be grateful for your efforts and acknowledge your growth.

Start to listen to your body and what it *needs* and not what it *wants*:

Your body is your best friend. If you treat it well, it will serve you well. It carries a lot of intelligence. Make use of it and start communicating with it. For example, the next time you are unsure if you should eat this thing or go for something else, ask your body what it needs to be fully nourished. And if you had a stressful day, the couch might be tempting, but going for a short walk might actually make you feel better. On another day, your energy level might be really low, and ditching the gym will be the better option. Do not do, or not do, anything out of laziness, but rather listen to your body's needs and act accordingly.

Forgive yourself for your past and future mistakes:

Self-love is a great term, but what is more practical (and eventually leads to self-love) is self-compassion. Imagine you are talking to your best friend and treat yourself with kindness. Instead of tearing yourself down for staying in this unhealthy relationship for too long or not sticking up for yourself, recognise that you have done your best and that this is enough. You are human. Human beings mess up and make mistakes. Know that you will continue to make mistakes but try to learn from them to avoid repeating making the same ones and know that you are still okay.

Give yourself a break:

Sometimes it is difficult to make a distinction between actually needing a break or looking for an excuse to not do something and procrastinate. If you are unproductive, even though you are trying to focus, or you are feeling unwell (physically, mentally and/or emotionally), give yourself a break. Use this time actively and instead of giving in to binge-watching your favourite TV series, why not try a new meditation, or going for a walk or taking a nap. Actively using the time to recharge your batteries and come back to feeling in tune with yourself will give you new energy to either achieve your goals or change them.

Make a list of things that make you feel good and things that make you feel uncomfortable:

Habits are created through the repetition of activities, meaning if you practise meditation for five minutes every day, you will develop a new habit after a few weeks. If you want to improve the quality of your everyday life, and incorporate more self-love, a great starting point might be looking at what you are doing right now, and how it affects you. Make a list of things that leave you feeling tense, depressed or low energy (e.g. eating junk food, drinking too much alcohol, consuming a lot of sugar, watching too much TV, overworking, skipping meals, the list goes on). Make another list of things beneficial to your wellbeing (e.g. being in contact with mother nature, taking time off work, watching a comedy film, attending a yoga class, conscious positive thinking, etc.). Now that you have written everything down and gained more awareness, make a conscious effort to exchange destructive behaviours with positive ones. And please enjoy a pizza once in a while without judging yourself – do it consciously and be aware that eating it every day leaves you with low energy.

Take care of your body and your mind:

Picture a car. If you don't put fuel into your car, it won't drive. If you give it the wrong fuel, it won't start either. The same goes for the body. Having a good diet and providing it with the right nutrients will keep it healthy. A car needs oil to keep the engine working, similar to how your muscles and ligaments want to be moved to stay fit and work smoothly. Just like your car, your body needs regular check-ups. The more you take care of your car throughout the year, the less likely it is to need big fixes. A working car is one you can use by getting behind the wheel, and navigating yourself from A to B. Imagine the driver is your mind and the car is your body. If your body has what it needs, you can focus on your mental wellbeing. Meditation is a great way to do this and helps to de-clutter and sharpen your mind.

Surround yourself with positive people:

Everyone has probably had the experience of meeting a friend and feeling completely drained afterwards. We, as humans, are empathic social beings, we are influenced by our surroundings and learn from others. Surrounding yourself with positive people will uplift you and bring you further in life. The more time you spend with them, the more you will adopt a positive mindset as well. Let yourself be uplifted and uplift others. Be(come) that person who, no matter what life throws at them, has a positive outlook on life and finds joy and gratitude in even the darkest of corners. Life is tough enough as it is, so make it fun and enjoy the ride.

Learn how to say "NO":

Remember, saying "no" to others is saying "yes" to yourself. Usually, people who say "yes" to everything and everyone are seeking validation from others. Once you give yourself this validation, you no longer need to do what others would like you to do. You are free from other reactions and can choose when to show up for others and know when you need to show up for yourself. You cannot give from an empty cup, so fill your own first and then share. You always have a choice. Choosing yourself is not selfish – it is actually the most sacred way of serving others. From this place, you can give freely, without feeling any resentment. Say "yes" to yourself always and know that by doing this, you are serving others as well.

Increase acceptance and compassion for yourself:

We ourselves tend to be our biggest critics. Next time that voice creeps up on you and tells you that you are not (good) enough, tell it to stop, breathe and show yourself some compassion by saying "I am enough". What would you say to a loved one after they messed up a job interview for example? Give yourself the same amount of understanding – hold space for yourself and accept yourself no matter what. Be your best friend and see the effort you put into preparing for that job interview, rather than the outcome.

Go to bed earlier:

Getting enough sleep is one thing; the other is going to sleep early. As we have biological tendencies to adapt our sleep pattern with that of the sun, we should ideally go to bed earlier and wake up early in the morning. Studies have found that we get less overwhelmed by pessimistic thoughts if we turn in early. Being well-rested lets us deal with emotions and problems better and helps us to stay calm in difficult situations. It also improves our productivity and sharpens our minds and helps with burning fat. Getting the right amount of sleep strengthens your immune system and makes you look fresh and healthy. Following the sun's movements also gives you the chance to catch more sunlight, which increases the brain's release of serotonin, making you happier and more comfortable in your skin.

Enhance joy and gratitude for life:

Have you watched a toddler exploring the world with joy and curiosity? Kids live in the present moment; their moods can go from crying to laughing in a second, and they embrace the joyful moments naturally. As adults, we often get caught up in our responsibilities and thinking about the future. Counting your blessings in bed before falling asleep by thinking of three things you are grateful for, connects you to the here and now and gets you out of a negative mindset. Laughing loudly brings joy, releasing endorphins and connecting you with your body. The road to self-love and compassion is one of joy and gratitude.

Take a long and relaxing bath with candles:

Sometimes after a long day at work, we want to come home, drop onto the couch and binge-watch our favourite TV series. And sometimes this can be exactly what you need, but often having more noise and visuals can lead to a sensory overload. In this case, running a bath for yourself might be more enriching. Create a loving atmosphere by lighting some candles, making some tea or pouring a glass of wine and even putting some gentle music on. Add some relaxing bath oil or Epsom salts (great if you have sore muscles) to the mix, and you are ready for some quality time alone. If you don't have a bathtub, you can also take a candlelit shower.

Enjoy the silence:

A lot of people live in big cities, which are constantly growing. More people in less space means more noise pollution. Exposure to loud noise can lead to high blood pressure, heart disease, sleep disturbances and stress. Considering this, investing in soundproof windows might be worthwhile. When you have some quiet time alone at home or you are out in nature for a walk, soak it all in and enjoy the quiet. Without outside noises to distract us, we are able to pay closer attention to what's going on inside and listen to what we need.

Spend more time with selected friends:

Surrounding ourselves with people who love and accept us for who we are makes us happy and boosts our self-worth. Instead of meeting new people all the time or people who leave you in an emotional limbo (like that person you have been dating who keeps vanishing on you), be aware of your worth and your time, and choose to spend it with those who value themselves and you. Connecting with loved ones, gives us a sense of belonging and makes us feel loved and appreciated. It's time to call that friend who you've been meaning to call for ages.

Meditate:

With so much content online, guided meditation is available all the time. As long as you have a smartphone, you can meditate anywhere. If you have not tried meditation yet, an in-person or online live course might be the right thing for you, as many offer a teacher or facilitator, so you can ask questions. There are also a lot of great apps and a wide range of meditations specialising in self-love. You can also take a few minutes in the morning after waking up, to breathe deeply (with your eyes closed), while telling yourself that you are enough and loved. I recorded a video about the basics of meditation, which you can view by going to my Instagram account and watching IGTV. Remember, that the energy flows to where you shift your awareness to.

Practise yoga:

Yoga is a holistic concept which improves your mind-body-soul connection. The physical exercises (*asanas*) strengthen and lengthen your body, breathwork (*pranayama*) calms down the mind and meditation (*dhyana*) connects you with your soul. In other words, yoga works out your body and supports a more relaxed outlook on life. From this place of wellbeing, it is only a short step to self-love and compassion.

Get regular health medical check-ups, blood tests, etc.:

A healthy body is the foundation of a healthy mind. When we are feeling unwell or we are physically ill, it very often takes a toll on our mental health as well. If you only eat junk food, you won't have much energy or feel good about yourself or in your own skin. Put a conscious effort into making your body the best possible place to live in for your mind and soul. When was the last time that you had a blood test? Get the recommended medical check-ups done and see a doctor if you feel like something is not right. Prevention and early detection are key and can save lives. As a cancer survivor, I am very aware of this and you should be too.

Tell yourself what you like about yourself:

The energy goes towards the focus. If you focus on what you dislike about yourself, you will probably feel pretty terrible. If instead you focus on the good and appreciate your good qualities, you will grow to like yourself more and more. Take a moment, sit or lay down and think about your positive traits. These can be physical or on a deeper level, referring to your nature or personality. Either say them out loud to yourself (for example: "I like your little button nose and your determination") or write them down in a list, so that the next time you doubt yourself, you can look at it and be reminded of the great stuff.

Stop looking for approval from others:

In times of social media, Photoshop and plastic surgery, it is easy to lose sight of what's actually important and base your self-worth on other people's opinions. Let's be honest here. There will be as many opinions about you as there are people in the world, meaning you will never get full approval from others – it's impossible! Instead, be grateful for who you are and how you show up in the world and validate yourself. You are the only one you spend 24/7 with, so treat yourself with kindness, especially when messing something up, and know that how you choose to show up says so much more about you, then any numbers on the scale. You won't be remembered for your perfect body, but rather for your passion and compassion.

Everyday do something that makes you happy:

Keep a list of things that spark joy for you or make you feel good. You can continually add to this list and do one of these things every day – especially when you 'don't have time'. This is when you most need your attention and something relaxing. Whether it is attending a yoga class, meditating, playing tennis or making yourself a delicious cup of cocoa with pure chocolate and spices, do one thing every day – and I repeat **every day** – to honour and treat yourself.

Make it a habit to make yourself happy. This will spark self-compassion and change your relationships as you stop relying on others for your happiness and create it yourself instead.

Don't take yourself too seriously:

Have you ever met someone you were attracted to and couldn't manage to get a word out of your mouth, or farted so loud in a yoga class everyone could hear it? We have all been in these situations. Instead of praying for the ground to open up and swallow you whole, have a laugh. Don't take yourself too seriously, but rather try to find the comedic moment in every situation. It is these kinds of embarrassing things that make us authentic and human.

Normalise making mistakes:

Remember that time you had a job interview, had no clue what you were talking about and were kicked out after the first round? I am pretty sure everyone's been in a situation of this kind, with your mind racing and feeling regret or, even worse, shame. Instead of judging yourself, pick up the pieces, shake it off and do it differently the next time around. Talk openly about your mistakes with your friends and family; take it off your chest and drop the shame around it because making mistakes is normal and is part of life. Don't overthink it. Instead, think of it as one of the best ways to learn and grow. Focus on what you could do better the next time, rather than torturing yourself and making new mistakes or repeating the same ones over and over.

Take actions in your life (don't be an actor, be the director of your life):

Often people are too afraid to take action as they might encounter rejection or failure. Instead, they stay in their safe four walls and dream about what life could be like. Yes, change is unpredictable. Yes, there are certain risks. And yes, outcomes are never completely predictable. And yet, this is where the most growth lies. Stepping out of your comfort zone and taking action opens new doors you might never have seen otherwise, and this is where the best things, where life, happens. Just having the courage to take action is empowerment and something we can be proud of, equalling higher self-worth. Don't just sit in the passenger's seat; take over the wheel and actively create the life you want for yourself. Which action will you take today?

Surround yourself with people who lift you up and motivate you:

The people you surround yourself with are a direct reflection of who you are or the person you are becoming. If you aspire to be a successful entrepreneur, surround yourself with others who are already there and who you can learn from. If your goal is to embody your inner truth, follow others who follow that path. The energy flows where attention goes, so consciously direct your attention towards what you want to achieve/who you want to become. Decide who to let into your energetic field and create a network with other like-minded people to support and uplift each other. There is a lot we can achieve by ourselves, but as a collective, we can go so much further.

Learn to enjoy your own company:

I love my own company and spending time by and with myself. In fact, I make it a priority to spend time with the number one person in my life – me. Having a strong and deep relationship with yourself creates a ripple effect and allows for deeper connections with others as well. If enjoying your own company is a fairly new concept to you, take a different approach to it. How would you treat your lover or your best friend? How would you spend your time with them? How would you show them your affection? What experience do you want them to have when they are spending time with you? And now, do all of these things for yourself, gift yourself with your own company, love and attention.

Take yourself out on dates – just you and the wonderful you:

This goes hand in hand with enjoying your own company. Part of this is to treat yourself the way you want others to treat you. If you want a partner who takes you out on amazing dates, be this partner for yourself first. This way, you improve your relationship with yourself and also get to truly enjoy being taken out by that special someone, as your needs are already met. Also, if you are in a long-term relationship or have kids, plan the occasional date with yourself. Cherish your own company and pamper yourself with the perfect date. Whether it is a hike in the great outdoors or a day at the spa, plan something that brings you joy and happiness. Having a certain regularity helps to maintain this even in the most stressful of times. Where will you take yourself on your next date?

Travel alone and be your own best friend:

Travelling alone is a powerful experience that combines many of the things already mentioned and inspires personal growth. Through solo travel, you learn self-reliance and take responsibility for your actions. You are forced to step out of your comfort zone and open up to new people and experiences. You will have to face loneliness and learn to enjoy time by yourself. If the thought of travelling alone makes you feel uneasy and you need some structure, book a surf camp or sign up for a course or an activity where you will meet people organically. It is your journey, so plan the trip you have always wanted to go on and give yourself the framework needed. For example, if you want to learn a new language, you might decide to do a work exchange to get to know some locals and practise the language. Or maybe you want to unwind and so you choose to go on a *vipassana* meditation retreat and sit in silence for several days. Whatever it is you have been wanting to do, start making plans and make it happen.

Write a list of all your accomplishments:

Criticising oneself comes easily to a lot of people. We tear ourselves down and hold onto our so-called 'failures'. Train your brain to see your growth and achievements instead. Make a list of all your accomplishments, writing down at least ten things that make you proud. And then put it up where you can see it multiple times a day. Repetition creates new neurological pathways. Next time the little, nagging voice of self-doubt whispers into your ear, tell it to stop and remember your achievements. Over time you will create a healthier self-image.

Let go of expectations:

One of the most painful experiences is having not just unfulfilled expectations but feeling them burst right in your face. When we expect something to work out a certain way or someone to meet our needs, we try to dictate an outcome and limit not just ourselves, but also the other person and eventually life itself. By setting expectations, we are creating blockages and hindering the natural flow. Life's gifts, more often than not, present themselves in ways we had never thought of. By limiting expectations (because realistically we will always have some at one point or another), you open yourself up to new pathways and possibilities. It is not just that you will end up less disappointed, but also find yourself being positively surprised. Make 'no expectations, no disappointments' your new mantra.

Embrace the idea that 'you are enough':

Nowadays we are bombarded with an endless number of pictures by (social) media that show us what 'perfect' looks like. No wonder so many of us have big insecurities, especially when it comes to body image. One way to boost your self-worth is to start following body positivity media accounts.

Surround yourself with realistic images and keep it real. From this place, it is a lot easier to accept yourself for who you really are. Tell yourself that you are enough, then meditate and sit with it, write it down and hang it up on the living room wall. Remind yourself of your 'enoughness' daily, until you have completely and fully internalised it, and then keep reminding yourself some more. And don't attach any conditions to it. You are enough, just as you are!

Try new things often, it will make you feel alive:

Trying out new things broadens your horizons and keeps life interesting. Feeling stuck is usually related to nothing changing on the outside, and nothing changing on the inside. As human beings, it is our desire to feel and to experience something new. Growth comes from new experiences too. Trying out new things is fun, it makes you a more diverse and interesting person and gives you more to talk about in conversations, but foremost it gives you that feeling of being alive. Make an effort to try out new things regularly. What have you been wanting to try for a long time? Just do it!

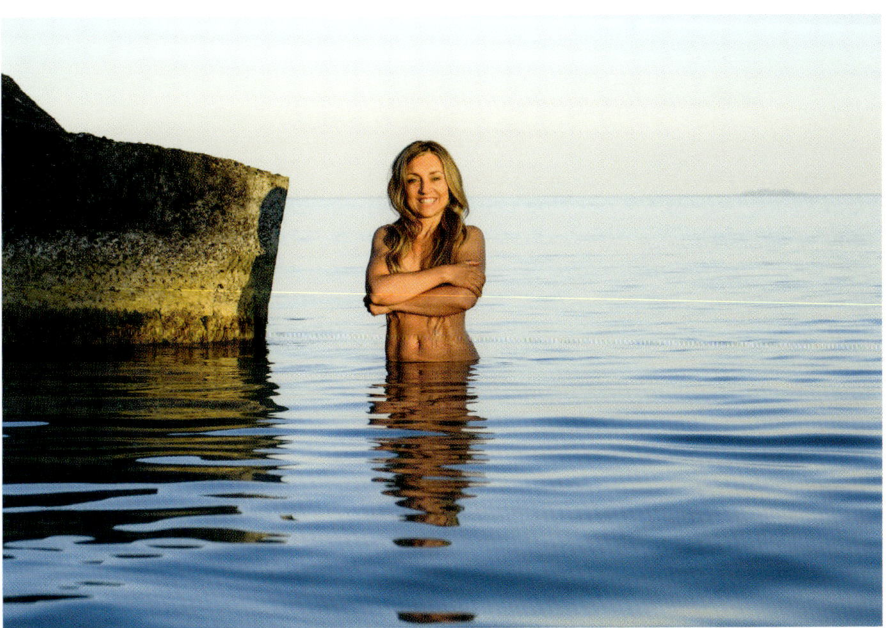

Be kind to others for no reason (and you will get positive energy back):

Being kind to others will make you feel good, as you will get positive energy in return. Try smiling at strangers for a day and see what happens. Even in big cities, where people often tend to be more suspicious, you will receive smiles back. Joy is infectious. If you are rather shy, you might want to be kind to others, but you might be a bit hesitant. Next time you see someone who could use your help, approach them and offer to help. This way, you are not just showing kindness towards others, but also coming out of your shell. The more positive energy you put out into the world, the more will come back to you.

Listen to that inner voice, trust your intuition:

The more you spend time with yourself and without distractions, the sharper your intuition, and the louder that inner voice will become. Having good intuition is like having a working compass with you when trying to navigate through stormy seas. If you have a feeling that something is wrong, stop ignoring it and listen to it instead, don't be afraid to say "no". The more you listen to that inner voice, the more aligned your life will become. Follow the joy, and do what feels right for you.

CHAPTER 14

Benefits Of Being Naked

*"Real beauty isn't about symmetry or weight or makeup. It's about looking life
right in the face and seeing all its magnificence
reflected in your own."*

– Valerie Monroe

Many recent studies have found several unexpected effects of nudism. First
and foremost, nudism is connected to a positive body image and overall
happiness – which is precisely what my message is all about. In this chapter,
I explore a more in-depth explanation of this.

What do the studies show?

Different studies show that participation in nudist activities leads to greater
overall life satisfaction. The main reason for this is that nudist participants
in the studies had a better body image and higher self-esteem, in comparison
to non-nudist participants.

I know what you are thinking: "These nudist people already have high
self-esteem and a positive body image. It's obviously not a problem for them
to be naked when other people are around. They are just comfortable like
this. Whereas people who have lower self-esteem and a rather bad body
image wouldn't even dare to be involved in any kind of nudist activity."And
yes, this does sound conclusive. But what we are missing here is that a
significant proportion of nudists are actually people who previously had
these issues themselves.

What changed?

Being naked together with other people is incredibly powerful in improving
your self-esteem and body image. It is very likely that at some point you will

be next to someone who has a 'flaw' that you feel like you have too. You feel ashamed about it, but the person next to you doesn't. Actually, no one next to you cares. So why would you? With these small questions, you already start to feel better about yourself.

The path to a greater body image and higher self-esteem:

For sure, it can take time to feel comfortable being naked. But you can slowly improve. And you will feel powerful with these small improvements you make. Which is how you can have greater life satisfaction too.

I know many people who would not have dared to get changed in a collective changing room, preferring to use the bathroom cubicle instead. After a few months, they started to get changed in the changing rooms and, at some point, they got used to it. They then showered with other people being around. And they also got used to it.

Eventually, these people are proud of their achievements. They feel stronger, and they are less scared. And they continue to change, permanently. They notice their flaws less and less. They start to focus on what matters. Some of them take part in nudist activities. Others don't. And it doesn't matter. In all instances, they have a better body image and higher self-esteem.

It is all about fear. You fear getting changed in front of others but realise that all the other people do it. You are afraid of being judged, but no one even notices what you are ashamed of.

It's okay if it takes you some time to realise it. It's okay if it takes you some time to get used to it. The key is to start this journey towards a healthier relationship with yourself and your body now. Here are some of the benefits of spending time in the nude.

You won't wake up tangled in your pyjamas:

Who hasn't experienced the discomfort of waking up in the morning, with your pyjamas halfway up your leg or your t-shirt almost strangling you? Sleeping naked means this era is officially over and you can feel free and move as you please while sleeping. If you are staying in a hotel, it's a good idea to have a bathrobe nearby in case the fire alarm goes off.

It prevents the risk of bacterial and yeast infections:

For anyone with a vagina, most of you will know how uncomfortable bacterial or yeast infections can be. The worst thing to do is to wear synthetic underwear. Sweating creates dampness, which is the perfect breeding ground for bacteria and yeast. Going 'commando' allows your vagina to breathe, preventing moisture and infections. Whether you are prone to infections or want to prevent them in the first place, wear cotton underwear or none at all.

Nudity enhances your relationships:

Showing yourself in the nude means showing yourself in all your glory and with all your insecurities. You literally drop the curtain and have nothing to hide behind. Doing this in your relationships helps you to see others for who they truly are and to be seen for who you are in return. It allows for more honest encounters and will make you more humble and allow you to connect with others on a deeper level.

Nudity frees you from social expectations:

Clothes are one way to show social status. When we wear expensive brands, we set ourselves apart from the rest. Usually, when we meet someone new, we judge them by their looks and outfit. Taking off our clothes means we are removing this barrier that separates us from one another, and instead we meet as human beings. We show up as we are in acceptance of each other.

Walking barefoot decreases the risk of Alzheimer's:

Remember the days when you were running around barefoot and carefree as a kid? Turns out, this is one of the best things to do to keep your brain young and agile. Going shoeless is officially recognised as an anti-Alzheimer's activity, that stimulates the brain to grow extra, efficient neuron connections through the sole sensation. Going barefoot does not just make you feel young at heart, but also rejuvenates your brain.

It's empowering to be looked at as a human being and not be judged on sex appeal or appearance:

We are all born naked and we all die naked – there is nothing we can take with us when leaving our bodies. Nudity is our natural state of being. Winning approval on social media will not build your self-esteem in the long run. Defining yourself through what others think of you is unhealthy and many posts portray toxic images of both femininity and masculinity. Showing up as who you are – naked – reverses this toxicity and improves self-confidence. Being regarded as a human being rather than as a sex object increases a sense of safety, especially for women.

Not wearing clothes gives you psychological release:

When a woman comes home after a long day of work she will often take off her bra, first thing. The bra for me is the embodiment of what we are doing daily. We put on a bra to help us present a social persona to the world. My recommendation is to completely strip off your clothes including your underwear and relax, once you are in a safe space (whether this is at home or a nudist event or another place). With time, this will become an automated process and you will relax (physically, mentally and emotionally) as soon as your clothes are off.

Nudity teaches you self-compassion:

Nudity on a physical level also makes it easier to be naked on other levels. Being naked means we are without any protection; we are vulnerable. Instead of criticising yourself over your imperfections, celebrate and create space for this vulnerability. By doing this, you open up a magic door to self-compassion. Give yourself approval and permission to be who you are, flaws and all. The more you are open and vulnerable with yourself, the more compassionate you will become.

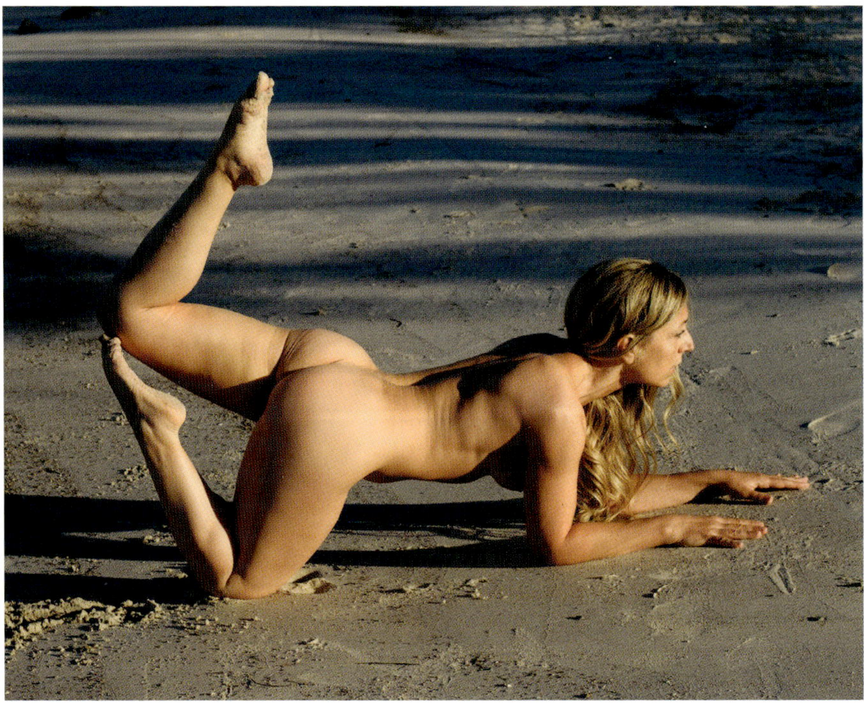

Self-acceptance:

As human beings, we are creatures of habit. Having some certainty gives us a sense of stability. Big changes can seem daunting, but you can also use this to your advantage. By just spending more and more time being nude, you can train yourself to accept your body with all of its imperfections. Make nudity your new norm by stripping off your clothes on a regular basis. I recommend looking at yourself in a mirror once in a while and complimenting yourself (tell yourself something like "I really like your long, gracious neck"). Focus on the good and forget about the rest. With time, you will learn to accept all of your body whatever shape or size you are.

Saves you money for laundry:

Due to the Covid-19 pandemic, in 2020 people spent a lot more time at home which led to a boom in nudity. People were naturally less bothered about getting dressed, especially in the summertime, as they were not leaving the house every day. Going nude means you are using fewer clothes, and that means doing less laundry. You might want to change your sheets a bit more regularly, but it will save on the rest. While spending your time being naked you are helping to improve your health, as well as saving money and supporting the environment.

Stronger bones and immune system:

Studies done by Harvard University have proven the beneficial effects of nudity on your health. Being exposed to the sun's rays increases your body's vitamin D levels. An optimal level of vitamin D equals a strong immune system, which helps you fight off viruses more easily and strengthens your bones. If you want to do something good for your health, try sunbathing in the nude (but avoid the midday heat to protect your skin).

Encourages breastfeeding by preventing mastitis infection:

A common issue faced by women who breastfeed is mastitis infection which can result in redness, swelling, breast pain and hotness. Restricting your breasts with a bra with pads to soak up any milk leakage is a good environment for infections to develop. Instead, spend some time topless to let the breasts air so that they dry and cracked nipples can heal. This will help prevent the infection in the first place and keep your breasts healthy for breastfeeding to continue without interruption.

It can spike male fertility:

Male fertility is declining. Wearing tight underwear and keeping your testicles warm contributes to this. Guys who wear boxers have a higher sperm concentration and higher sperm count than those wearing tighter styles. There is also a correlation between bad sleep and lower semen quality. Sleeping nude helps to stay cool and increases sleep quality providing a double win for male fertility. Time to get under the sheets in your birthday suit.

You will discover muscles you didn't know you had:

Most of us will be rather used to seeing our faces or checking our outfits in the mirror. Being naked allows us to see what we usually don't. You might find a muscle you didn't know you had or realise just how toned your calves are after spending the whole of summer outside, going for hikes and bike rides. Be open to noticing and discovering new things about your body when shedding your clothes.

No bikini lines:

In the summertime many of us spend a lot of time outside, exposing ourselves to the sun. As clothes are cut differently, people with lighter skin tones end up with an uneven tan – not to mention those spots where the sun doesn't reach. By ditching the swimwear and any other types of clothes, you avoid this and give your body the chance to produce more vitamin D.

Discover and treat skin conditions:

Nudity offers multiple benefits for the skin. On the one hand, there is nothing rubbing against it and no itchiness caused by certain materials. Your skin can breathe and heal itself better (if you, for example, suffer from any skin conditions). Being naked also helps in preventing serious skin issues developing and makes spotting them, or other visible health problems such as new lumps, easier.

You will live a happier life:

Studies have shown a link between nudity and higher levels of happiness. Compared to people who spend their days dressed, naturists have a better connection and are more content with their bodies. There is a correlation between how long one has been practising nudism and their happiness levels, meaning the more time you spend in the nude, the happier you will become.

No clothes, no stigma:

We live in a highly sexualised world. With social media and internet access basically everywhere, pornography is available at the snap of a finger. If nakedness was the norm and a common experience, as it once was for our ancestors, this unhealthy interest in pornography would be considerably lessened. While some people can watch porn now and then and not suffer any ill effects, many people, from pre-teens upwards, are drawn to watching pornography compulsively. This leads to an unrealistic view of sex and intimacy, impairing the viewer's ability to become aroused by a real-life sexual partner. Being comfortable naked enables a more relaxed way for the genders to live side-by-side and appreciate each other as people. Nudity has the power to change our society for the better.

Kids will grow up without shame:

Most neuroses and phobias have their root in childhood. Children growing up in nude households become unperturbed by the human body later in life, which can lead to higher psychological strength as well. Growing up in a family where nudity is the norm makes a greater contribution to a high body self-concept than one's race, gender or the area that one lives in. Let's teach our future generations self-confidence, by normalising nudity, and erasing the shame around it.

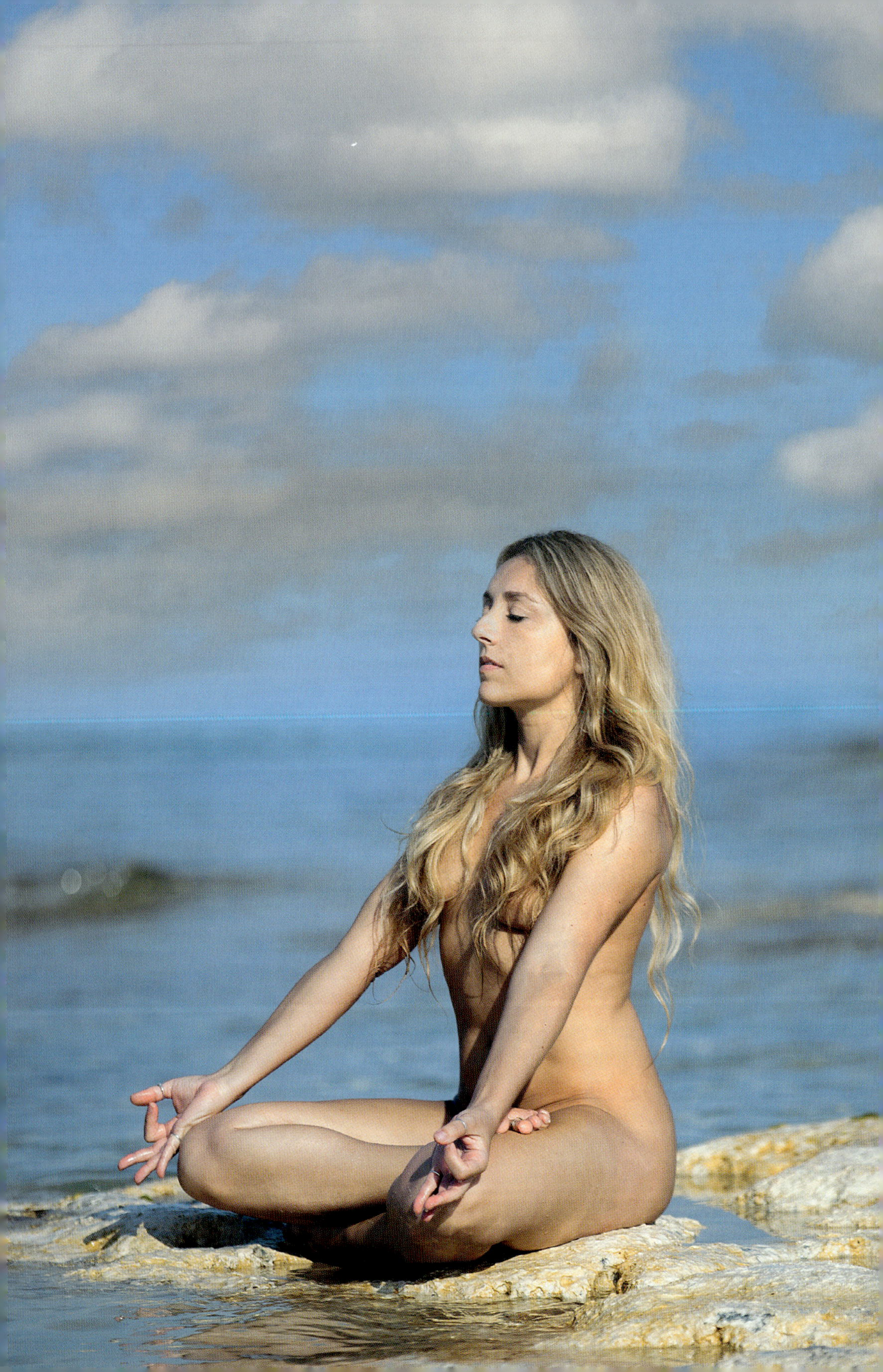

CHAPTER 15

How To Reconnect With Yourself

"When people go within and connect with themselves, they realize they are connected to the universe and they are connected to all living things."
– Armand Dimele

It is easy to get caught up in the stress of daily life. When there is a lot going on on the outside, it can be difficult to keep the focus on the inside. When the external world becomes overwhelming, we should all return to the internal world and retreat to the basics. Just like anything else in life, practise is key. The more often you (re)connect with your body, the more deeply rooted you will be in yourself, making you more resilient to stress and less likely to get out of balance in the first place. Maybe you already have some tools and know-how to reconnect with yourself, or maybe this is completely new to you. Either way, you will find some inspiration in my go-to tips below. Investing in a grounding practice and making this part of your daily routine can make a huge difference in the quality of your everyday life. Consistency is key here, making five minutes a day to practise, is often more effective than spending an hour on it once a week. Trying out different things will give you a better understanding of your needs and a bigger insight into what works for you and what doesn't.

Daily gratitude ritual:

Gratitude boosts your mental and physical health, improves your self-esteem and fosters resilience. Counting your blessings also has a positive effect on your sleep quality. Gratitude furthermore enhances empathy and reduces aggression. Being grateful towards others also improves your social life. You can practice gratitude in different ways. You can set up a little altar with things that bring you joy and remind you of the good in your life with pictures of family and friends, motivational quotes, a little statue of a god or goddess (I have Ganesh on my altar), some incense, a candle, essential oils, crystals, flowers, etc. Go there in the morning and say your 'thank yous' for everything and everyone you have in your life (for example, be grateful for the roof over your head, the food on the table, all your great friendships, a rewarding profession that brings you joy and so on). Having this little corner in your home will remind you to be grateful. You can also take a few minutes after waking in bed in the morning and say out loud what you are grateful for. This will set the tone for the day and help you to stay centred and grounded and, most of all, positive.

Learn to live in the present moment:

Your breath is your anchor to the present moment. When stressed, your breath becomes quick and shallow, while breathing slowly and deeply calms down the nervous system. When you feel yourself worrying about the future or reliving the past, conscious breathing is one way of coming back to the present moment. Also realising when you are drifting off, and making the decision to focus on what's right in front of you, will help you to be in the here and now. When getting up in the morning set the intention to be fully present and make the most of what is happening around you. There is nothing to worry about when staying in the present and focussing on the current task. Remember, you can't change the past, but you can ruin the present by worrying about the future.

Positive affirmations:

The origin of the word affirmation comes from the Latin word *affirmare*, which means 'to make steady, strengthen'. Thoughts turn into words which turn into actions. By thinking positively and reassuring yourself through affirmations, new neurological pathways are created in your brain. Positive thoughts can literally raise the level of feel-good hormones. Your brain cannot differentiate between what is true and what is not, and thoughts create emotions. The more often you repeat something, the more it will become reality. Use this tool to break through negativity and replace it with positivity.

Here are a few examples of positive affirmations: I am the architect of my life, I build its foundation and choose its contents; I know I can accomplish anything I set my mind to; I forgive myself for not being perfect because I know I'm human; I respect myself; I believe everything works out for the best; I know, accept and am true to myself. You can find many more affirmations on the internet or you can just create your own.

Tech detox:

Have you noticed how many people are glued to their phones nowadays? It always amazes me to see everyone on their phone, while on the train or the bus. Hardly anyone is paying attention to their surroundings or looking at others. And have you tried making eye contact with strangers? People will give you a weird look like you are crazy. Just as a fast cleanses your body, a tech detox cleanses your mind. Going on holiday is the perfect time to temporarily say goodbye to social media and the like.

In your daily life, setting certain limitations like no phones at the dinner table will improve your home life, connect you to the present and bring you closer together with your loved ones. Set yourself a small goal and try it out, starting with leaving your phone at home for one day or one full weekend.

Mantras:

A mantra is a short sound, word or phrase in Sanskrit used for meditation purposes by repeating it over and over again. This repetition helps to keep the mind focussed and stay present. They are considered sacred and they focus your intention and calm your mind. The most well-known example is "Om", which is said to be the first sound heard at the creation of the universe. When pronouncing it fully, the energy should rise up from your pelvic floor all the way up through the crown of your chakra. Attending yoga classes, you will learn many more mantras to reconnect with yourself.

Law of attraction:

Using the law of attraction is a great starting point for change. By thinking about what it is that you truly desire in your life, you put your energy towards it. For example, if you want to start a new job, picture yourself having a new job and focus on what it feels like rather than what the job exactly looks like. The next step is to take simple actions, meaning looking at different job offers before applying for some. While going through the application process, come back to how it feels to have a new job, without getting attached to the outcome of one job interview. Your thoughts will pave the way to slowly make big changes and live a fulfilled life. Practising the law of attraction will help you to attract what you deeply want in your life.

Intuitive eating:

I believe there is so much truth in the saying, "You are what you eat". Remember, just like a car, your body works in similar ways in the sense of, if you use the wrong fuel, the motor won't start, and the car won't move. The more you nourish your body and the more you provide it with (the right) nutrients, the more energetic and happier you will be. Your body is a miracle in what it daily does for you and it knows very well what it needs as a fuel. If you eat a lot of sugar and processed foods, your body gets used to these additives and loses its natural intelligence a bit. Once you detox it of sugar and too much salt, you will be able to communicate with your body and ask it what it needs. If you have a craving for avocado toast, then listen to your body and give it to it. Your body is your natural compass in the world of eating. Forget diets, just learn how to hear your body's voice and nourish yourself accordingly.

Mindful eating:

With the hectic lifestyle many of us lead nowadays, taking time to eat is often a luxury. Or seems like one. As an alternative to junk food, an Italian journalist named Carlo Petrini started the Slow Food Movement in Italy back in 1986 which supports local food and traditional cooking. He also encourages taking your time to eat and developing your sense of taste. Being Italian myself, I think this movement is fantastic and the perfect foundation for mindful eating. It starts when you buy your foods (try a local market instead of the supermarket to get local and seasonal produce) and continues when preparing your food. Take your time to cook and do it with love. Imagine how delicious and nourishing the dish will be while preparing it. Once your food is ready, sit down, take a deep breath and breathe in the smells of what you prepared (this will also enhance the taste of it) and slowly take the first bite. Take your time to chew and fully experience the taste of it. This will bring you right back into the here and now. Enjoy!

Get in touch with old (childhood) friends:

Kids have this special lightheartedness. They are completely immersed in the present moment and can go from crying to laughing within a few seconds. The more social interactions we have, the more often we laugh throughout the day. Reconnecting with old friends from your childhood can bring out your inner child and make you remember all the fun you had back in the day. Lifelong friendships are special and don't come along that often. Treasure the memories you have, call an old friend of yours, spend a day being silly together and reconnect with your inner child.

Sports:

Working out is good for your heart and improves your mental and physical health. It also can provide you with an outlet for stress and negativity. When exercising hard you cannot afford to go through negative thinking patterns over and over again. You need to stay focussed and concentrate on your breath and posture to avoid injury and collapsing from too little oxygen. In short, exercising is the perfect way to get out of your head and into your body. Completing a tough workout will also give you a feeling of accomplishment and improve your self-worth. Next time you get caught up in unhealthy thinking patterns, grab your running shoes and hit the pavement.

Journaling:

Journaling provides the perfect outlet for stuck emotions and uncomfortable feelings. Your journal is your safe space where you can open up completely without anyone judging you. You can either have a topic to write about (like how you want to show up today) or set your alarm and free write. Even just five minutes of it will have a beneficial effect. Getting your thoughts down on paper means getting them out of your head. If you struggle to relax at night and to go to sleep, take your journal and write down everything that's on your mind. Then close it and put it away. You may continue to think about certain decisions tomorrow, but for now, it is time to rest.

Walking outside (leave your phone at home):

Nature has a proven positive effect on you. Just looking at a picture of a forest calms the nervous system and releases tension. When you get overwhelmed with life or you are exhausted and need a break, grab your comfy shoes and go outside. Maybe you are lucky enough to live next to the ocean or are surrounded by mountains. If you live in a city, go to the nearest park, walk around and look up to the trees. To get the most out of this, leave your phone at home or put it into flight mode. You won't need Google Map and your Instagram followers can wait until tomorrow for your next 'story'. This is your break – celebrate it.

Music:

Music triggers emotions. When you hear a song you used to listen to as a child, it brings back memories and lets you relive the situation. Music is a powerful tool. When you are agitated, find some relaxing music, put your headphones on and immerse yourself in it. Maybe lay down and breathe deeply or get up and gently move your body.

Spa day/treatments:

Many of us neglect ourselves when caught up in the stress of daily life. When this happens, setting aside time to pamper yourself can bring you closer to reconnecting with your body. If you had a stressful week, book a massage to release the built-up tension or create an at-home spa and relax with candlelight.

Healing from old family traumas:

No family is perfect, even if it might look great from the outside. The people who raise us have a massive impact on us and influence our (future) relationships. We fall in love with what we know, meaning that we will probably reproduce that difficult relationship with a parent in a close partnership as it is familiar. Working through old family traumas clears up a lot of space, frees you from old (behavioural) patterns and opens you up for new types of relationships. Investing in yourself is one of the most sustainable things to do. Whether you have a family member you haven't spoken to in years and want to call them or you are thinking about seeing a psychotherapist, pick up the phone now and take action.

Hanging out with pets:

I absolutely love animals, especially dogs. Spending quality time with animals has a positive impact on your mood and health. It reduces stress and calms the nervous system. Pet owners (especially ones with a close relationship with their pets) are generally happier, more trusting and less lonely than people without pets. Pets often sense when you don't feel well and come over to be with you. Having a pet in your life can give you a sense of purpose and belonging, and they will love you unconditionally.

Don't reach for your phone first thing in the morning (create your own healthy morning routine):

Smartphones make it is easy to be reachable and on social media 24/7. Many people reach for their phone first thing after waking up. What you do in the first few minutes when awakening in the morning sets the tone for the rest of the day. Do you check your emails, appointments or maybe Facebook and TikTok? You might want to rethink this behaviour. I recommend having your phone turned off or on flight mode during the night to improve your sleep quality and to keep it slightly out of reach when in bed. Maybe even consider getting an old-school alarm clock to check the time, in case you wake up during the night. When you wake up, resist the urge to grab your phone right away and replace this habit with a more beneficial one. Create your own, healthy routine. Meditation first thing and visualising the events of the day ahead is a great way to start. This will set you up for success and you can always check your phone later on.

Baking:

Whether or not you have baking experience, it is a productive activity, and the lockdown period provided the perfect time to learn it. With baking, you have an immediate outcome. It might be tasty or sometimes not even edible, in which case you can give it another go. Getting out of your head and working/creating something with your own hands can give you a sense of achievement. And afterwards, you get to eat (and ideally enjoy) the product as well. Bake something delicious and enjoy it slowly.

Help someone else:

What you put out into the world is what you will receive. The more positivity you exude and the more good you do, the more goodness will come your way. When you are in a place where you can give, do so freely. It will make you feel good by giving you an extra sense of purpose and expanding your focus to others. For example, you can make a donation to an organisation which you support. Let's give each other a helping hand and lift up one another.

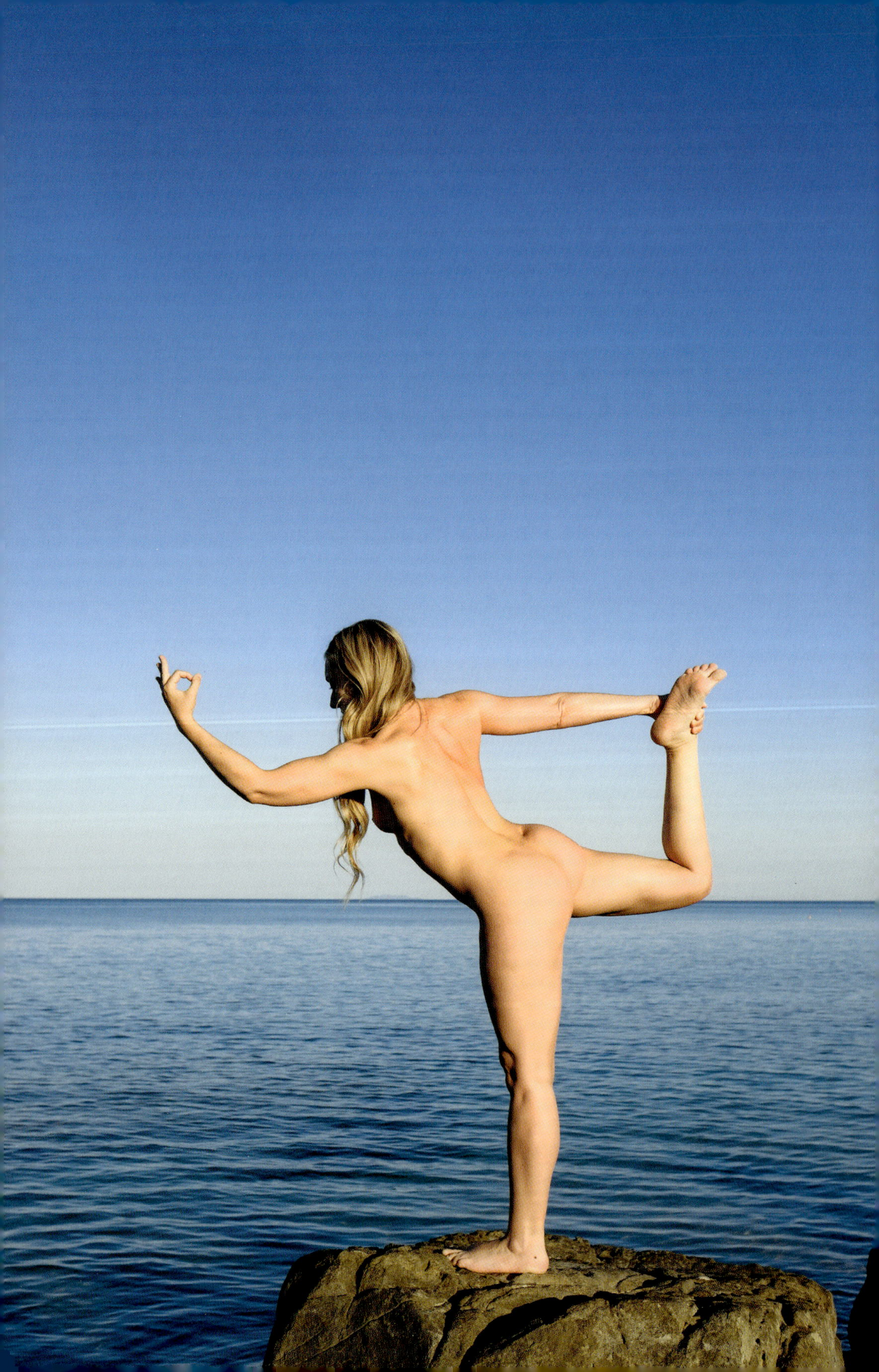

PART THREE

Beginners' Yoga Guide

Surya Namaskar A

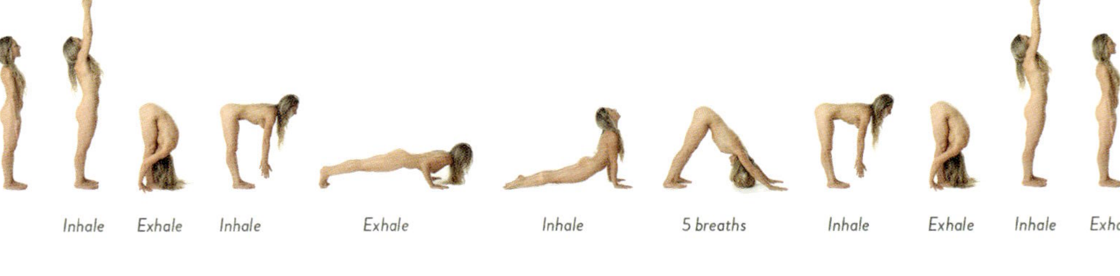

Surya Namaskar B

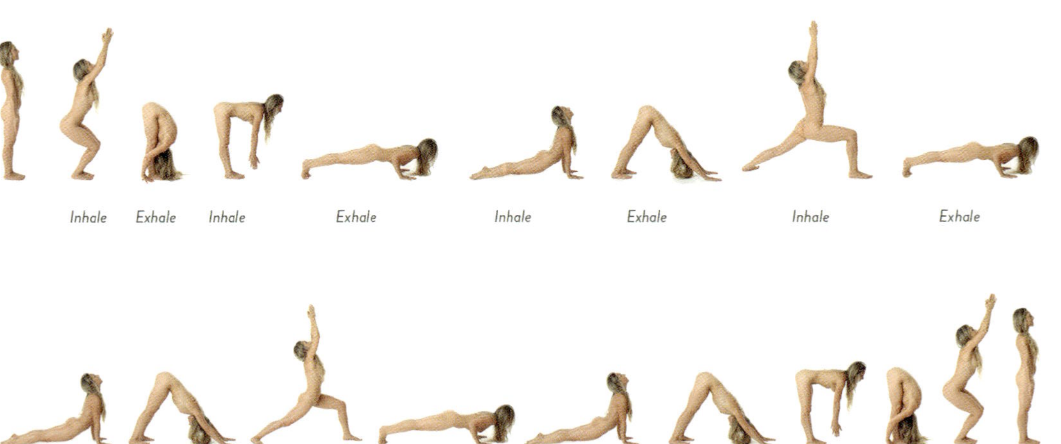

Chapter 16

Sun Salutations A & B

"As I bow to the sun, I bow to myself and give gratitude to my body, my health and wellbeing, the universe and all of its creations. I welcome life and light and let go of everything that does not serve me anymore."

(Unknown)

Whether you are new to yoga or are already an advanced practitioner, Sun Salutations (*Surya Namaskar* in Sanskrit) are a great way to get started with yoga and keep your practice consistent. In only 20 minutes you can experience improvements in your health and wellbeing.

The Sun Salutations consist of different components which make up a *vinyasa* – a series of movements used between poses in Ashtanga, Vinyasa and Power yoga. They are very often used as a warm-up program as they build up heat in the body. Practising Sun Salutations regularly increases blood flow to the muscles and lengthens them, which improves the range of motion throughout the whole body.

Each pose is coordinated with the breath (inhale to extend, and exhale to bend), which helps to create a meditative flow. In Ashtanga yoga, we differentiate between *Surya Namaskar A* and *B*. Always breathe in and out through your nose in all Sun Salutations and let your breath lead your movement.

Sun Salutation Surya Namaskar A

Sanskrit name: *Surya Namaskar* (SOOR-yah nah-mahs-KAHrah)

Meaning: Sun Salutation

Skip if: You have a hernia

You suffer from high blood pressure or coronary artery disease

You have a weak heart or have had a stroke

You are on your period, listen to your body's needs and proceed accordingly

You suffer from back conditions (please seek proper advice before commencing *Surya Namaskar* A & B)

1. Mountain Pose

Sanskrit name: *Tadasana* (tah-DAHS-anna)

Meaning: *Tada* = mountain, *asana* = posture/pose

These movements are usually used to start off an asana practice. Before starting, I recommend taking a moment to ground yourself. Deepen your breath and focus on your feet. Feel the connection to the ground beneath and pay attention to your weight distribution. Do you have more weight on one foot or in a certain part of your feet? Scan your whole body and feel the sensations that arise.

Benefits from practising Mountain Pose regularly:

Strengthens thighs, knees and feet

Helps to improve posture

Firms up the abdomen and buttocks

Sciatica relief

Skip if: You suffer from insomnia or low blood pressure

How to practise:

Step 1: Stand with your feet parallel to each other, big toes slightly touching.

Step 2: Lift your toes, spread them and lower them back down to the ground, rock sideways and back and forth, distribute your weight evenly and come to a standstill.

Step 3: Bring your pelvis into a neutral position by picturing a bucket of water and finding the perfect position where the water doesn't overflow.

Step 4: Bring your head back a bit and make a slight double-chin to align it with your spine, then let your arms hang beside your body.

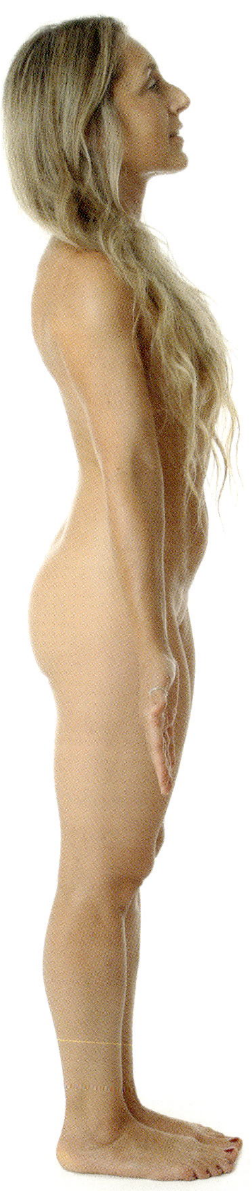

Mountain Pose

Tip: Spending some extra seconds on getting the right posture in this pose is worth the effort as this is your starting point for your Sun Salutations and many other asanas.

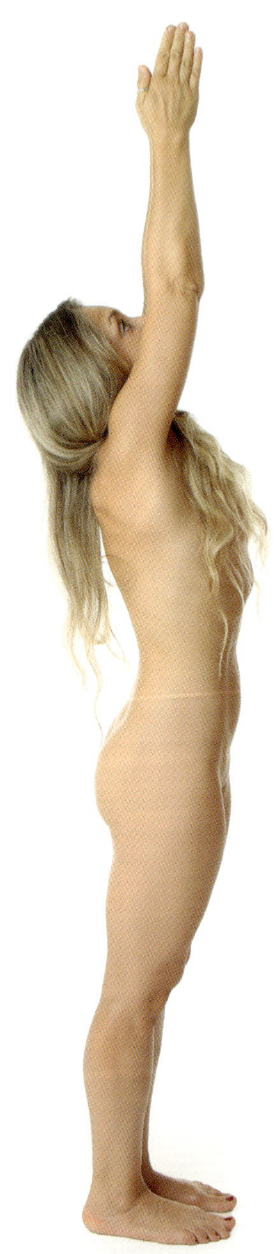

Upward Salute

2. Upward Salute

Sanskrit name: *Urdhva Hastasana* (oord-vah hahs-TAHS-anna)

Meaning: Raised hands pose: *urdhva* = raised (or upward), *hasta* = hand, *asana* = posture/pose

Benefits from practising Upward Salute regularly:

Helps to relieve back pain

Improves fatigue and indigestion

Stretches front body

Stretches shoulder

Skip if: You suffer from shoulder or neck injuries

How to practise:

Step 1: From Mountain Pose *(Tadasana)*, raise your arms out to the side and all the way up towards the ceiling.

Step 2: Bring the palms of your hands together and give yourself a good stretch by reaching up as high as you can.

Step 3: Next, squeeze your buttocks (for stability) and lean back ever so slightly, gaze upwards.

Tip: Don't try to keep your shoulders down as you raise your arms up high, let them move organically with your arms.

3. Standing Forward Fold

Sanskrit name: *Uttanasana* (OOT-tan-AHS-ahna)

Meaning: Stretched posture: *uttana* = intense stretch/straight, *asana* = posture/pose

Benefits from practising Standing Forward Fold regularly:

Calms the nervous system and aids in the relief of stress, fatigue and mild anxiety; Aids in relieving menopause symptoms

Stimulates the liver and kidneys and supports good digestion

Strengthens thighs, stretches hamstrings, calves and hips

Beneficial for asthma, high blood pressure, headaches and insomnia

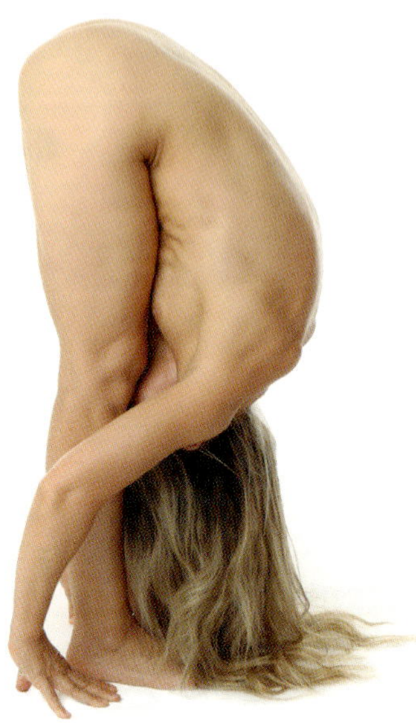

Standing Forward Fold

Skip if: You have a back injury

How to practise:

Step 1: From Upward Salute *(Urdhva Hastasana)*, fold from the hips and bend forward, arms lowering down to the ground.

Step 2: If possible, place the palms of your hands flat on the ground in front of your feet, alternatively let them hang and reach for the ground.

Step 3: Relax your neck and let your head hang heavy.

Tip: When folding forward make sure to avoid locking your knees; if necessary, bend your knees ever so slightly.

4. Standing Half-Forward Bend

Sanskrit name: *Ardha Uttanasana* (are-dah oot-tan-AHS-anna)

Meaning: *Ardha* = half, *uttana* = intense stretch/straight, *asana* = posture

Benefits from practising the Standing Half-Forward Bend regularly:
Stretches the front torso, improves posture, strengthens the back

Skip if: You have a back injury and be cautious with neck problems

How to practise:

Step 1: From Standing Forward Fold *(Uttanasana)*, press your fingertips against the floor and lift up your sternum, away from the ground, you can alternatively place the palms of your hands on your shins or keep your arms vertical to the floor.

Step 2: Bring your spine parallel to the floor, your head is an extension of it.

Tip: Microbend your knees to avoid locking them.

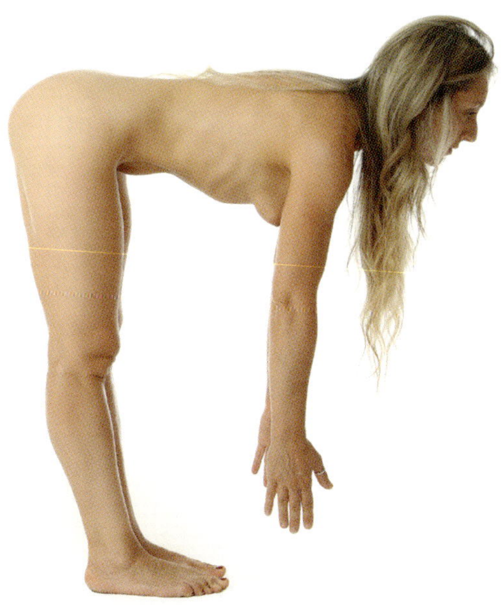

Standing Half-Forward Bend

5. Four-Limbed Staff Pose

Sanskrit name: *Chaturanga Dandasana* (chaht-tour-ANG-ah don-DAHS-anna)

Meaning: *Chaturanga* = four limbs, *danda* = staff (refers to the spine, the central 'staff' or support of the body), *asana* = posture/pose

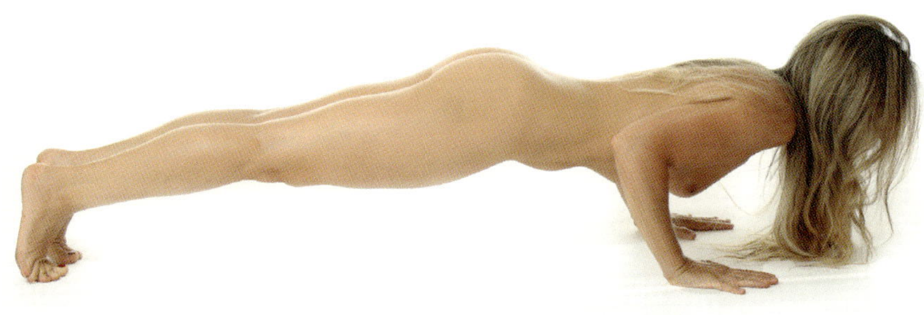

Four-Limbed Staff Pose

Benefits from practising the Four-Limbed Staff Pose regularly:

Builds strength in the arms and wrists

Firms up your abdominal muscles

Skip if: You have carpal tunnel syndrome

How to practise:

Step 1: From Standing Half-Forward Bend, *(Ardha Uttanasana)* bring the palms back down to the ground and step back into a plank position.

Step 2: Bring your hands below your shoulders, squeeze your buttocks and activate your abdominal muscles to release tension from your spine, make sure your whole body is in one straight line.

Step 3: Slowly lower your torso and your legs down to the ground, hugging your ribs with your elbows (keep them close to your body throughout).

Step 4: Make sure not to collapse in your shoulders, keep them activated and the space between the shoulder blades broad, look forward.

Tip: If you are a beginner or have not built up enough strength yet, lower your knees down onto the floor.

6. Upward Facing Dog Pose

Sanskrit name: *Urdhva Mukha Shvanasana* (OORD-vah MOO-kah shvon-AHS-anna)

Meaning: *Urdhva* = up/upwards, *mukha* = face, *shvana* = dog, *asana* = posture/pose

Benefits from practising Upward Facing Dog Pose regularly:

Strengthens the spine, arms and wrists
Stretches the front torso and lungs
Shapes the buttocks
Stimulates the abdominal organs
Aids in relieving fatigue, mild depression and sciatica

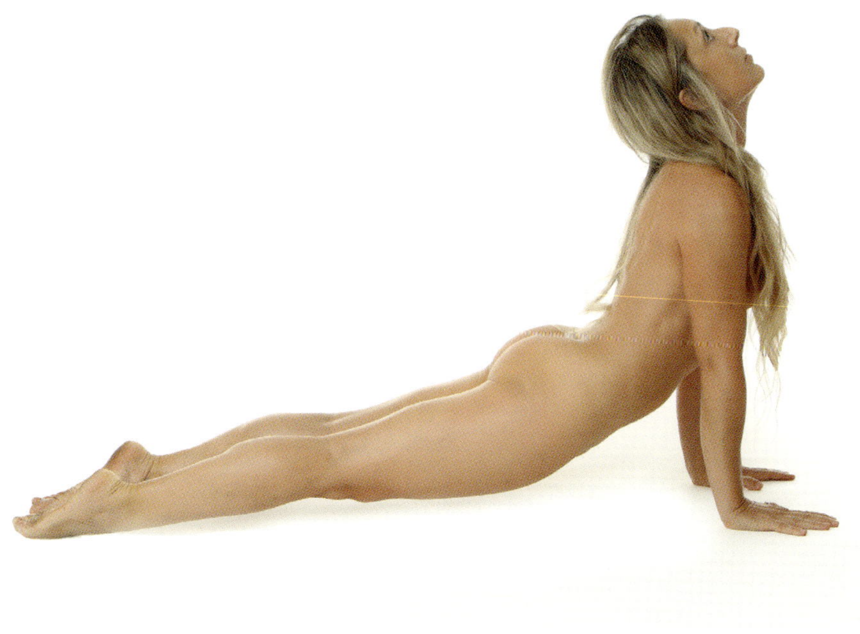

Upward Facing Dog Pose

Skip if: You have an injured back or carpal tunnel syndrome

How to practise:

Step 1: From Four-Limbed Staff Pose *(Chaturanga Dandasana)*, push the floor away with the palms of your hands.

Step 2: Bring your shoulders back and down, away from your ears and open your chest.

Step 3: Squeeze your buttocks really hard to avoid pressure on your lower back and imagine you are holding a yoga block with your thighs (or actually put one between them and squeeze).

Step 4: Lift the pubis off the ground, only your hands and your legs should be touching it.

Tip: Microbend your elbows to protect your joints.

7. Downward Facing Dog Pose

Sanskrit name: *Adho Mukha Shvanasana* (AH-doh MOO-kah shvah-NAHS-anna)

Meaning: *Adho* = downward, *mukha* = face, *shvana* = dog, *asana* = posture/pose

Benefits from practising Downward Facing Dog regularly:

Relieves headaches, stress, fatigue and mild depression

Helps shoulders, hamstrings, calves and hands to stretch

Strengthens arms and legs

Aids in relieving menopause symptoms as well as menstrual discomfort

Supports a healthy digestion

Beneficial for asthma, sciatica and sinusitis

Skip if: You suffer from carpal tunnel syndrome or diarrhoea

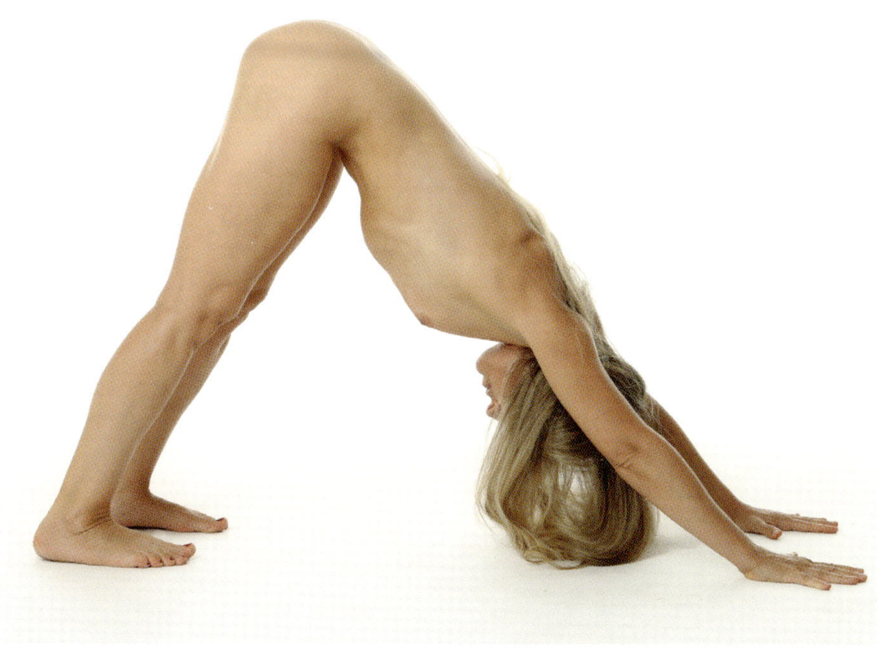

Downward Facing Dog Pose

How to practise:

Step 1: From Upward Facing Dog *(Urdhva Mukha Shvanasana)*, press your hands into the ground, put your head down to look backwards and lift your torso up towards the ceiling.

Step 2: Push back, lower your heels down on the ground (or near it), keep your legs straight (without locking them); if necessary, bend them slightly.

Step 3: Lift your sitting bones towards the ceiling and activate your abdominal muscles.

Step 4: Push the floor away with your hands and keep your head between your arms (don't let it hang, it should be aligned with your spine).

Tip: Don't get obsessed with getting your feet all the way down to the ground; instead, focus on having a good form.

8. Standing Half-Forward Bend

Sanskrit name: *Ardha Uttanasana* (are-dah oot-tan-AHS-anna)

Meaning: *Ardha* = half, *uttana* = intense stretch/straight, *asana* = posture

Benefits from practising the Standing Half-Forward Bend regularly:

Stretches the front torso

Improves posture

Strengthens the back

Skip if: You have a back injury and be cautious with neck problems

How to practise:

Step 1: From Downward Facing Dog *(Adho Mukha Shvanasana)*, look forward between your hands and step forward on your mat one foot at a time, you can place the palms of your hands on your shins or keep your arms vertical to the floor.

Step 2: Bring your spine parallel to the floor, your head is an extension of it.

Tip: Microbend your knees to avoid locking them.

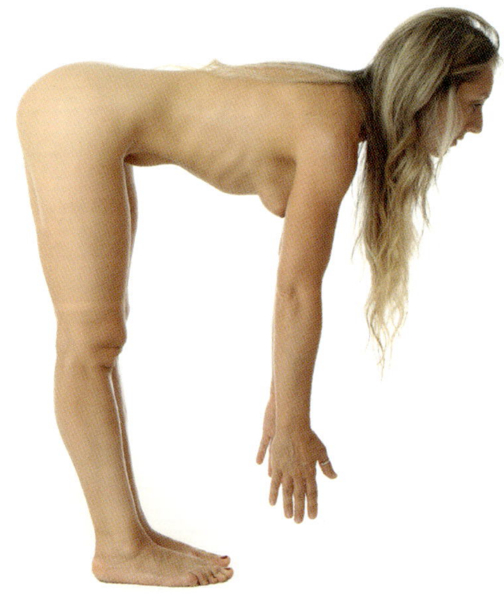

Standing Half-Forward Bend

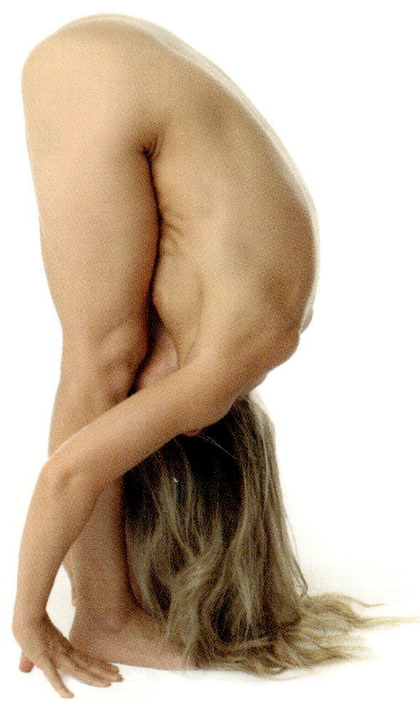

Standing Forward Fold

9. Standing Forward Fold

Sanskrit name: *Uttanasana* (OOT-tan-AHS-ahna)

Meaning: Stretched posture: *uttana* = intense stretch/straight, *asana* = posture/pose

Benefits of practising Standing Forward Fold regularly:

Calms the nervous system, relieving stress, fatigue and mild anxiety

Stimulates the liver and kidneys and supports good digestion

Strengthens thighs, stretches hamstrings, calves and hips

Aids in relieving menopause symptoms

Beneficial for asthma, high blood pressure, headaches and insomnia

Skip if: You have a back injury

How to practise:

Step 1: From Standing Half-Forward Bend *(Ardha Uttanasana)*, fold from the hips and bend forward, arms lowering down to the ground.

Step 2: If possible, place the palms of your hands flat on the ground in front of your feet, alternatively let them hang and reach for the ground.

Step 3: Relax your neck and let your head hang heavy.

Tip: When folding forward make sure to avoid locking your knees; if necessary, bend your knees ever so slightly.

10. Upward Salute

Sanskrit name: *Urdhva Hastasana* (oord-vah hahs-TAHS-anna)

Meaning: Raised hands pose: *urdhva* = raised (or upward), *hasta* = hand, *asana* = posture/pose

Benefits of practising Upward Salute regularly:

Helps to relieve back pain

Improves fatigue and indigestion

Stretches front body

Stretches shoulder

Skip if: You suffer from shoulder or neck injuries

How to practise:

Step 1: From Standing Forward Fold *(Uttanasana)*, raise your arms out to the side and all the way up towards the ceiling.

Step 2: Bring the palms of your hands together and give yourself a good stretch by reaching up as high as you can.

Next, squeeze your buttocks (for stability) and lean back ever so slightly, gaze upwards.

Tip: Don't try to keep your shoulders down as you raise your arms up high, let them move organically with your arms.

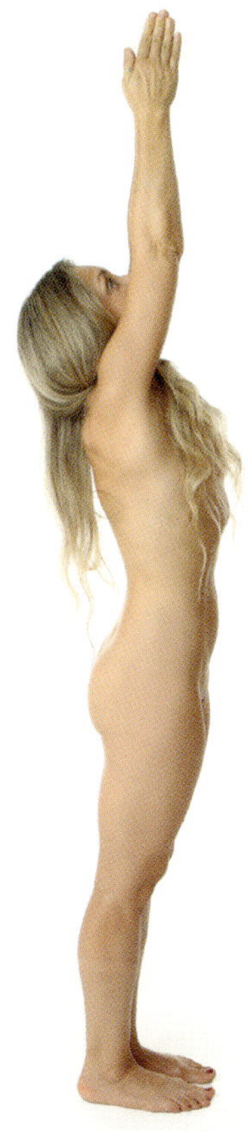

Upward Salute

11. Mountain Pose

Sanskrit name: *Tadasana* (tah-DAHS-anna)

Meaning: *Tada* = mountain, *asana* = posture/pose

Deepen your breath and focus on your feet. Feel the connection to the ground beneath and pay attention to your weight distribution. Do you have more weight on one foot or in a certain part of your feet? Scan your whole body and feel the sensations that arise.

Benefits of practising Mountain Pose regularly:

Strengthens thighs, knees and feet

Helps to improve posture, firms up the abdomen and buttocks

Relieves sciatica

Skip if: You suffer from insomnia or low blood pressure

How to practise:

Step 1: Stand with your feet parallel to each other, big toes slightly touching.

Step 2: Lift your toes, spread them and lower them back down to the ground, rock sideways and back and forth, distribute your weight evenly and come to a standstill.

Step 3: Bring your pelvis into a neutral position by picturing a bucket of water and finding the perfect position where the water doesn't overflow.

Step 4: Bring your head back a bit and make a slight double-chin to align it with your spine, then let your arms hang beside your body.

Tip: At the end of your Sun Salutation A *(Surya Namaskar A)* program, spend at least 5 minutes lying on the ground on your back in Corpse Pose *(Shavasana)* to enjoy and benefit from deep relaxation.

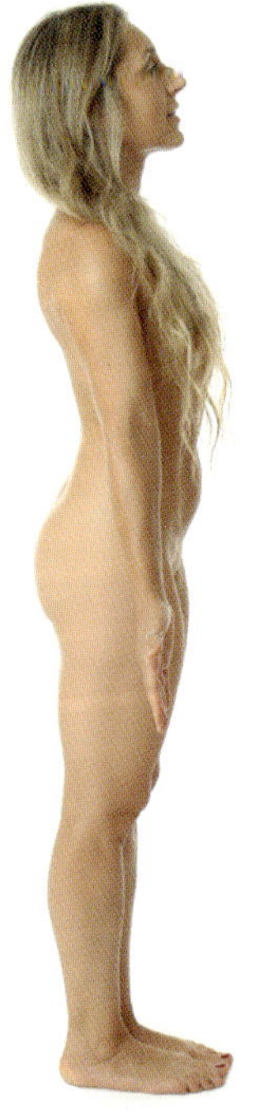

Mountain Pose

Sun Salutation Surya Namaskar B

Once you are confident doing *Surya Namaskar A*, you can start adding *Surya Namaskar B* to your routine. The A series is the perfect preparation, as it offers gentler exercises. The B variation of the program creates more heat, with the added chair pose, and is the extension of the A version. It consists of more asanas than *Surya Namaskar A* and is more challenging for your muscles as well as your cardiovascular system.

Once you are familiar with *Surya Namaskar B,* it provides a great base, to which you can start adding more asanas.

1. Mountain Pose

Sanskrit name: *Tadasana* (tah-DAHS-anna)

Meaning: *Tada* = mountain, *asana* = posture/pose

Benefits from practising Mountain Pose regularly:

Strengthens thighs, knees and feet

Helps to improve posture

Firms up the abdomen and buttocks

Relieves sciatica

Skip if: You suffer from insomnia or low blood pressure

How to practise:

Step 1: Stand with your feet parallel to each other, big toes slightly touching.

Step 2: Lift your toes, spread them and lower them back down to the ground, rock sideways and back and forth, distribute your weight evenly and come to a standstill.

Step 3: Bring your pelvis into a neutral position by picturing a bucket of water and finding the perfect position where the water doesn't overflow.

Step 4: Bring your head back a bit and make a slight double-chin to align it with your spine, then let your arms hang beside your body.

Tip: Spending some extra seconds on the right posture in this pose is worth the effort as this is your starting point for your Sun Salutations and many other asanas.

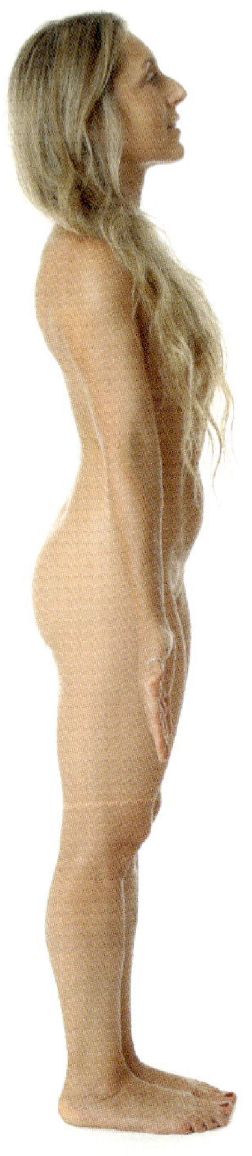

Mountain Pose

2. Chair Pose

Sanskrit name: *Utkatasana* (OOT-kah-TAHS-anna)

Meaning: Wild or difficult posture/power posture, *utkata* = wild/intense/powerful/fierce/difficult, *asana* = posture/pose

Benefits of practising Chair Pose regularly:

Strengthens ankles, thighs, calves, feet and spine

Stretches shoulders and chest, stimulates abdominal organs, diaphragm and heart

Skip if: You suffer from insomnia or low blood pressure

How to practise:

Step 1: From Mountain Pose *(Tadasana)*, raise your arms up until they align with your spine, palms facing inwards and bend your knees.

Step 2: Lower your buttocks down slowly, activate your core.

Step 3: Keep the lower back long by taking your tailbone down towards the ground and in towards your pubis.

Tip: Squeeze your knees together for extra support in this posture.

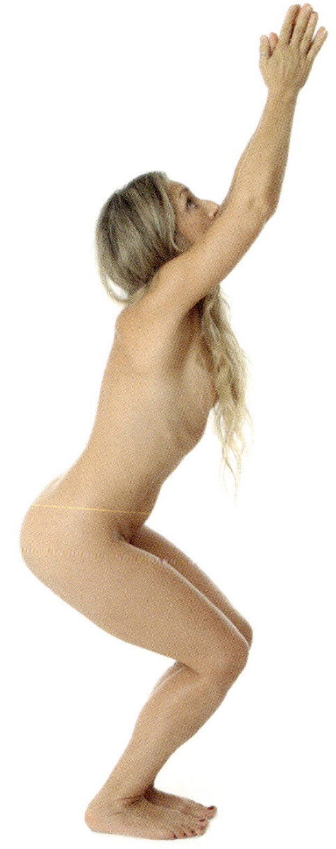

Chair Pose

3. Standing Forward Fold

Sanskrit name: *Uttanasana* (OOT-tan-AHS-ahna)

Meaning: Stretched posture, *uttana* = intense stretch/straight, *asana* = posture/pose

Benefits from practising Standing Forward Fold regularly:

Calms the nervous system

Aids in the relief of stress, fatigue and mild anxiety

Stimulates the liver and kidneys and supports good digestion

Strengthens thighs

Stretches hamstrings, calves and hips

Aids in relieving menopause symptoms

Beneficial for asthma, high blood pressure, headaches and insomnia

Skip if: You have a back injury

How to practise:

Step 1: From Chair Pose *(Utkatasana)*, fold from the hips, straighten your legs and bend forward, arms lowering down to the ground.

Step 2: If possible, place the palms of your hands flat on the ground in front of your feet, alternatively let them hang and reach for the ground.

Step 3: Relax your neck and let your head hang heavy.

Tip: When folding forward, make sure to avoid locking your knees; if necessary, bend your knees ever so slightly.

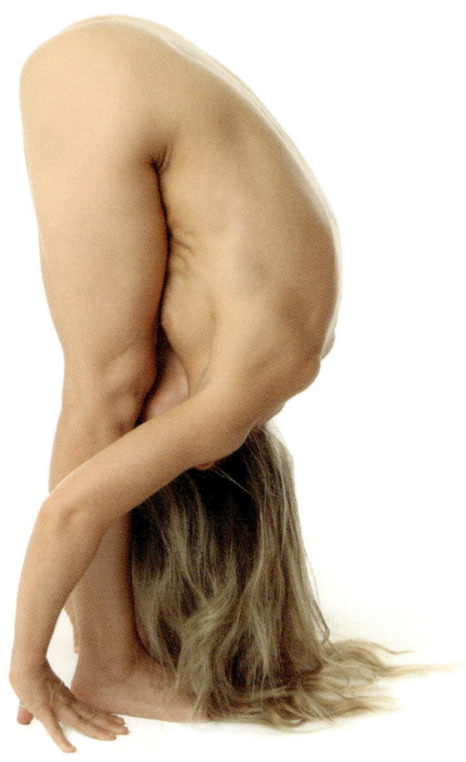

Standing Forward Fold

4. Standing Half-Forward Bend

Sanskrit name: *Ardha Uttanasana* (are-dah oot-tan-AHS-anna)

Meaning: *Ardha* = half, *uttana* = intense stretch/straight, *asana* = posture/pose

Benefits from practising Standing Half-Forward Bend regularly:

Stretches front torso

Improves posture

Strengthens back

Skip if: You have a back injury and be cautious with neck problems

How to practise:

Step 1: From Standing Forward Fold *(Uttanasana)*, press your fingertips against the floor and lift up your sternum, away from the ground; alternatively, place the palms of your hands on your shins, or just keep your arms vertical to the floor.

Step 2: Bring your spine parallel to the floor, your head is an extension of it.

Tip: Microbend your knees to avoid locking them.

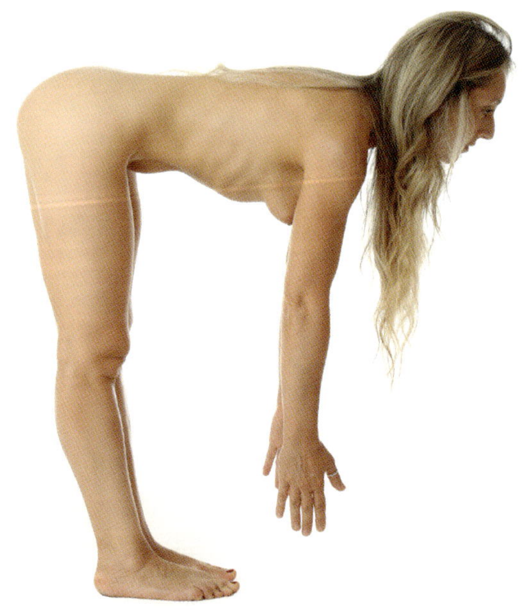

Standing Half-Forward Bend

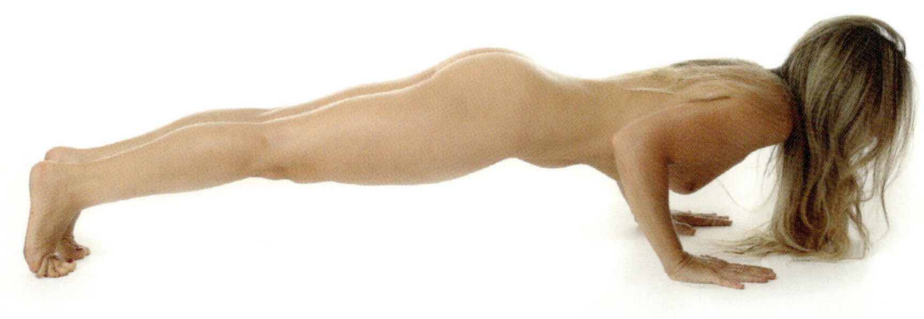

Four-Limbed Staff Pose

5. Four-Limbed Staff Pose

Sanskrit name: *Chaturanga Dandasana* (chaht-tour-ANG-ah don-DAHS-anna)

Meaning: *Chaturanga* = four limbs, *danda* = staff (refers to the spine, the central 'staff' or support of the body), *asana* = posture/pose

Benefits from practising Four-Limbed Staff regularly:

Builds strength in the arms and wrists and firms up abdominal muscles

Skip if: You have carpal tunnel syndrome

How to practise:

Step 1: From Standing Half-Forward Bend *(Ardha Uttanasana)*, bring the palms back down to the ground and step back into a plank position.

Step 2: Bring your hands below your shoulders, squeeze your buttocks and activate your abdominal muscles to release tension from your spine; make sure your whole body is in one straight line.

Step 3: Slowly lower your torso and your legs down to the ground, hugging your ribs with your elbows (keep them close to your body throughout).

Step 4: Make sure not to collapse in your shoulders, keep them activated and the space between the shoulder blades broad, look forward.

Tip: If you are a beginner or have not built up enough strength yet, lower your knees down onto the floor.

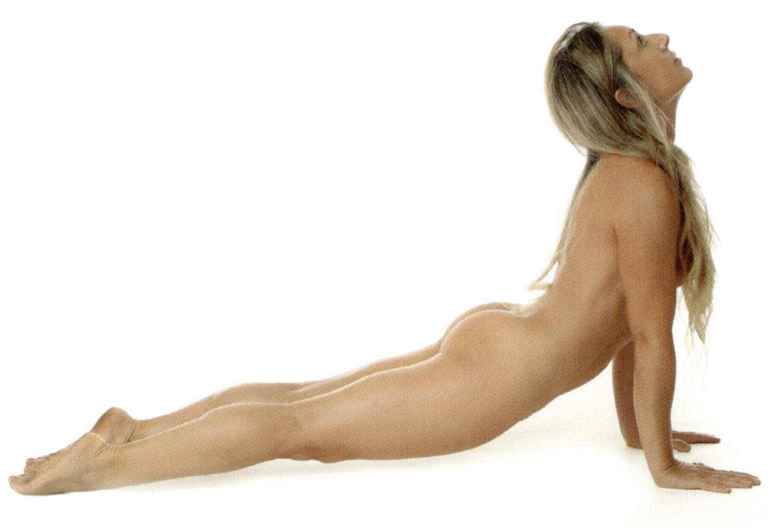

Upward Facing Dog Pose

6. Upward Facing Dog Pose

Sanskrit name: *Urdhva Mukha Shvanasana* (OORD-vah MOO-kah shvon-AHS-anna)

Meaning: *Urdhva* = up/upwards, *mukha* = face, *shvana* = dog, *asana* = posture/pose

Benefits from practising Upward Facing Dog regularly:

Shapes buttocks, strengthens the spine, arms and wrists

Stretches the front torso and lungs, stimulates abdominal organs

Aids in relieving fatigue, mild depression and sciatica

Skip if: You have an injured back or carpal tunnel syndrome

How to practise:

Step 1: From Four-Limbed Staff Pose *(Chaturanga Dandasana)*, push the floor away and lean into the palms of your hands.

Step 2: Bring your shoulders back and down, away from your ears and open your chest.

Step 3: Squeeze your buttocks really hard to avoid pressure on your lower back and imagine you are holding a yoga block with your thighs (or actually put one between them and squeeze).

Step 4: Lift the pubis off the ground, only your hands and your legs should be touching it.

Tip: Microbend your elbows to protect your joints.

7. Downward Facing Dog Pose

Sanskrit name: *Adho Mukha Shvanasana* (AH-doh MOO-kah shvah-NAHS-anna)

Meaning: *Adho* = downward, *mukha* = face, *shvana* = dog, *asana* = posture/pose

Benefits from practising Downward Facing Dog regularly:

Relieves headaches, stress, fatigue and mild depression

Stretches the shoulders, hamstrings, calves and hands

Strengthens arms and legs

Aids in relieving menopause symptoms as well as menstrual discomfort

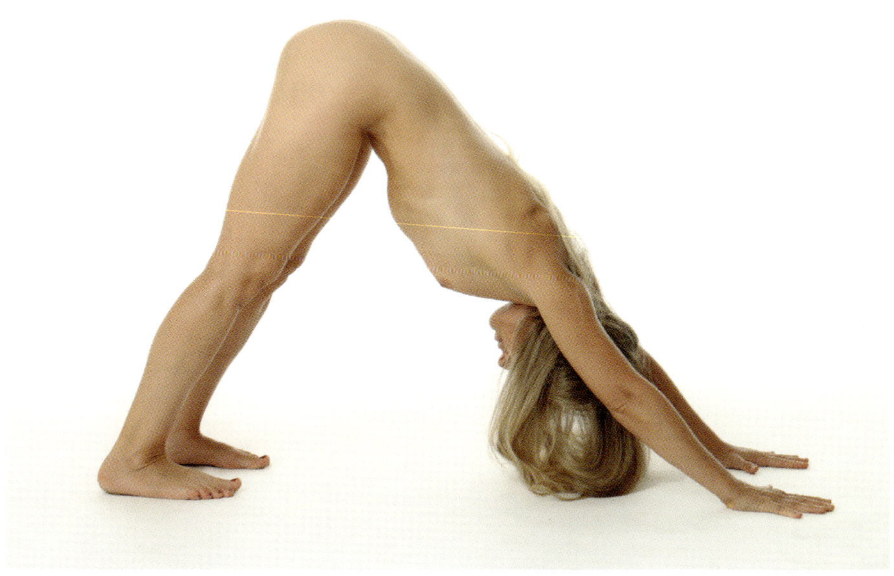

Downward Facing Dog Pose

Supports healthy digestion

Beneficial for asthma, sciatica and sinusitis

Skip if: You suffer from carpal tunnel syndrome or diarrhoea

How to practise:

Step 1: From Upward Facing Dog Pose (*Urdhva Mukha Shvanasana)*, press your hands into the ground and lift your torso up towards the ceiling.

Step 2: Push back, lower your heels down on the ground (or near it), keep your legs straight (without locking them); if necessary, bend them slightly.

Step 3: Lift your sitting bones towards the ceiling and activate your abdominal muscles.

Step 4: Push the floor away with your hands and keep your head between your arms (don't let it hang, it should be aligned with your spine).

Tip: Don't get obsessed with getting your feet all the way down to the ground; instead, focus on having a good form.

8. Warrior I Pose Right Leg

Sanskrit name: *Virabhadrasana* I (veer-ah-bah-DRAHS-anna)

Meaning: *Virabhadra* = warrior/hero, *asana* = posture/pose

Benefits from practising Warrior I Pose Right Leg:

Beneficial for sciatica

Stretches the chest, lungs, shoulders, neck and belly

Strengthens the arms, shoulders and back muscles

Strengthens and stretches the thighs, calves and ankles

Skip if: You suffer from high blood pressure or heart problems

How to practise:

Step 1: In Downward Facing Dog Pose *(Adho Mukha Shvanasana)*, raise your right leg and step it forwards in between your hands (if necessary, adjust the foot afterwards).

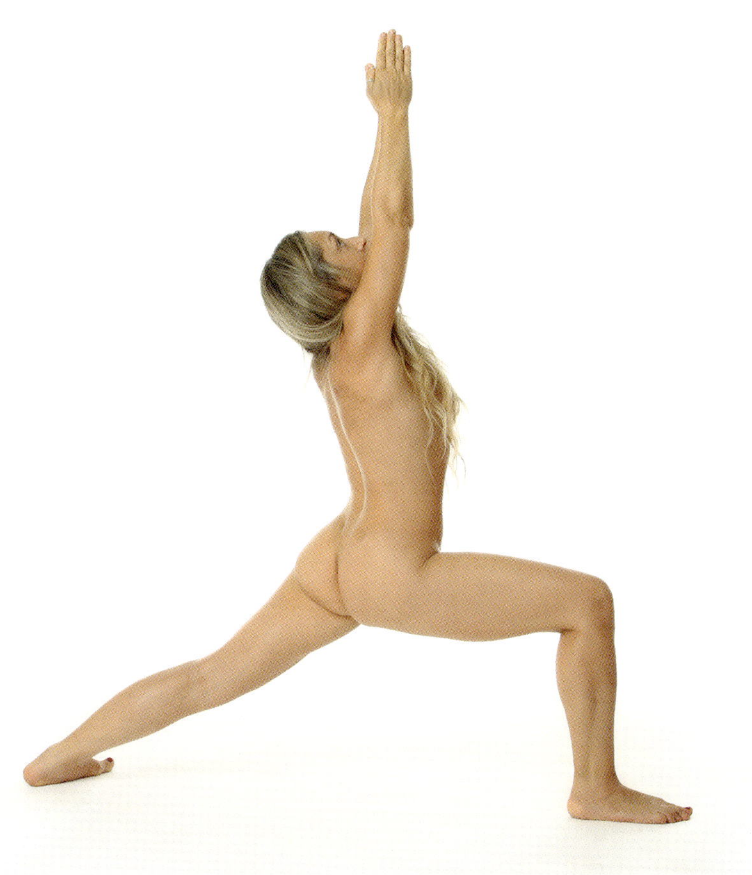

Warrior 1 Pose Right Leg

Step 2: Turn your left foot 45 degrees outwards, align your heels.

Step 3: Bring your hands together, raise your arms above your head.

Step 4: Turn your torso, chest pointing to the front, hips square, front knee in line with your front heel.

Step 5: Tilt your pelvis ever so slightly, long lower back.

Tip: Keep your head in a neutral position to avoid neck problems.

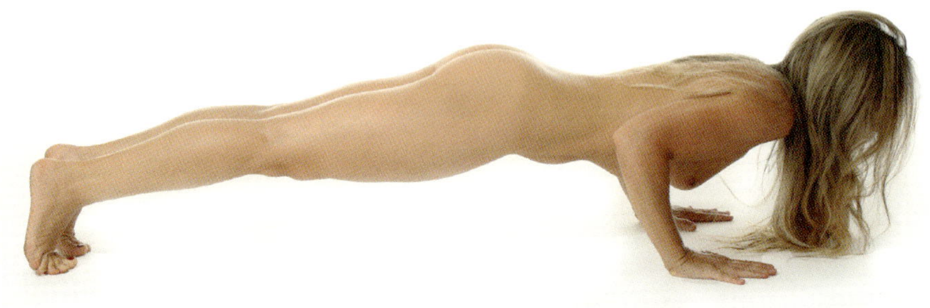

Four-Limbed Staff Pose

9. Four-Limbed Staff Pose

Sanskrit name: *Chaturanga Dandasana* (chaht-tour-ANG-ah don-DAHS-anna)

Meaning: *Chaturanga* = four limbs, *danda* = staff (refers to the spine, the central 'staff' or support of the body), *asana* = posture/pose

Benefits from practising the Four-Limbed Staff Pose regularly:

Builds strength in the arms and wrists

Firms up your abdominal muscles

Skip if: You have carpal tunnel syndrome

How to practise:

Step 1: From Warrior 1 Right Leg *(Virabhadrasana I)*, bring the palms back down to the ground and step back into a plank position.

Step 2: Bring your hands below your shoulders, squeeze your buttocks and activate your abdominal muscles to release tension from your spine, make sure your whole body is in one straight line.

Step 3: Slowly lower your torso and your legs down to the ground, hugging your ribs with your elbows (keep them close to your body throughout).

Step 4: Make sure not to collapse in your shoulders, keep them activated and the space between the shoulder blades broad, look forward.

Tip: If you are a beginner or have not built up enough strength yet, lower your knees down onto the floor.

10. Upward Facing Dog Pose

Sanskrit name: *Urdhva Mukha Shvanasana* (OORD-vah MOO-kah shvon-AHS-anna)

Meaning: *Urdhva* = up/upwards, *mukha* = face, *shvana* = dog, *asana* = posture/pose

Benefits from practising Upward Facing Dog Pose regularly:
Shapes the buttocks, strengthens the spine, arms and wrists
Stretches the front torso and lungs, stimulates the abdominal organs
Aids in relieving fatigue, mild depression and sciatica

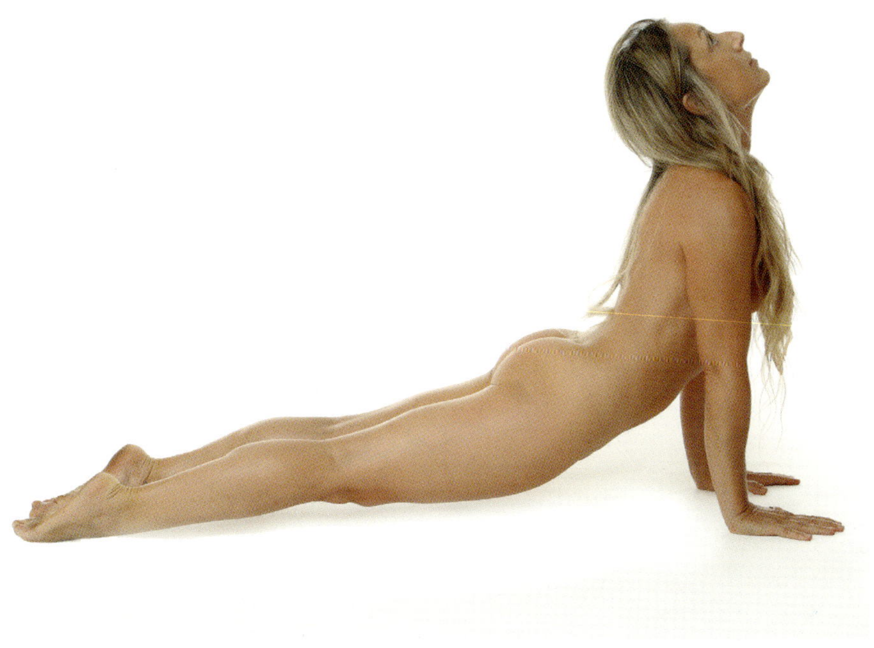

Upward Facing Dog Pose

Skip if: You have an injured back or carpal tunnel syndrome

How to practise:

Step 1: From Four-Limbed Staff Pose (*Chaturanga Dandasana)*, push the floor away and lean into the palms of your hands.

Step 2: Bring your shoulders back and down, away from your ears and open your chest.

Step 3: Squeeze your buttocks really hard to avoid pressure on your lower back and imagine you are holding a yoga block with your thighs (or actually put one between them and squeeze).

Step 4: Lift the pubis off the ground, only your hands and your legs should be touching it.

Tip: Microbend your elbows to protect your joints.

11. Downward Facing Dog Pose

Sanskrit name: *Adho Mukha Shvanasana* (AH-doh MOO-kah shvah-NAHS-anna)

Meaning: *Adho* = downward, *mukha* = face, *shvana* = dog, *asana* = posture/pose

Benefits from practising Downward Facing Dog regularly:

Relieves headaches, stress, fatigue and mild depression

Stretches shoulders, hamstrings, calves and hands

Strengthens arms and legs

Aids in relieving menopause symptoms as well as menstrual discomfort

Supports a healthy digestion

Beneficial for asthma, sciatica and sinusitis

Skip if: You suffer from carpal tunnel syndrome or diarrhoea

How to practise:

Step 1: From Upward Facing Dog *(Urdhva Mukha Shvanasana)*, press your hands into the ground and lift your torso up towards the ceiling.

Step 2: Push back, lower your heels down on the ground (or near it), keep your legs straight (without locking them); if necessary, bend them slightly.

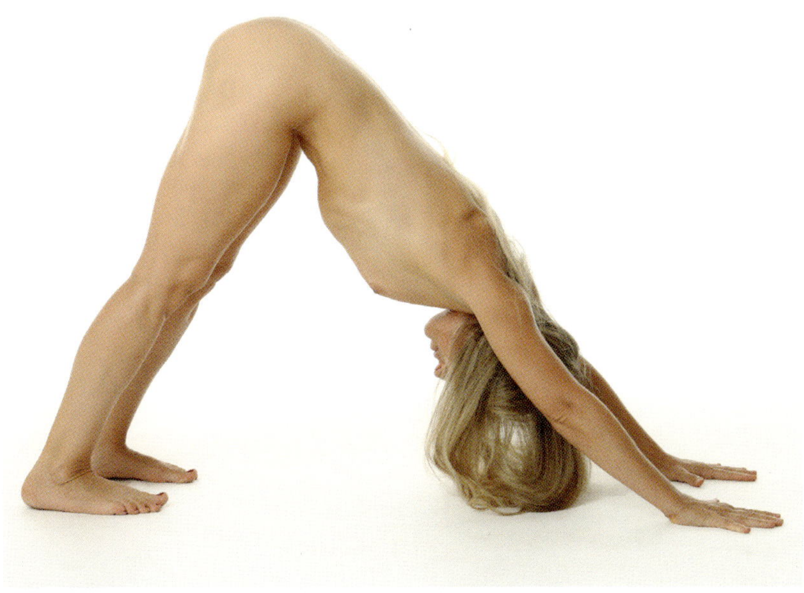

Downward Facing Dog Pose

Step 3: Lift your sitting bones towards the ceiling and activate your abdominal muscles.

Step 4: Push the floor away with your hands and keep your head between your arms (don't let it hang, it should be aligned with your spine).

Tip: Don't get obsessed with getting your feet all the way down to the ground; instead, focus on having a good form.

12. Warrior 1 Pose Left Leg

Sanskrit name: *Virabhadrasana* I (veer-ah-bah-DRAHS-anna)

Meaning: *Virabhadra* = warrior/hero, *asana* = posture/pose

Benefits of practising Warrior I Pose Left Leg:

Beneficial for sciatica

Stretches chest, lungs, shoulders, neck and belly

Strengthens arms, shoulders and back muscles

Strengthens and stretches thighs, calves and ankles

Skip if: You suffer from high blood pressure or heart problems

How to practise:

Step 1: In Downward Facing Dog *(Adho Mukha Shvanasana)*, raise your left leg and step it forwards in between your hands (if necessary, adjust the foot afterwards).

Step 2: Turn your right foot 45 degrees outwards, align your heels.

Step 3: Bring your hands together, raise your arms above your head.

Step 4: Turn your torso, chest pointing to the front, hips square, front knee in line with your front heel.

Step 5: Tilt your pelvis ever so slightly, long lower back.

Tip: Keep your head in a neutral position to avoid neck problems.

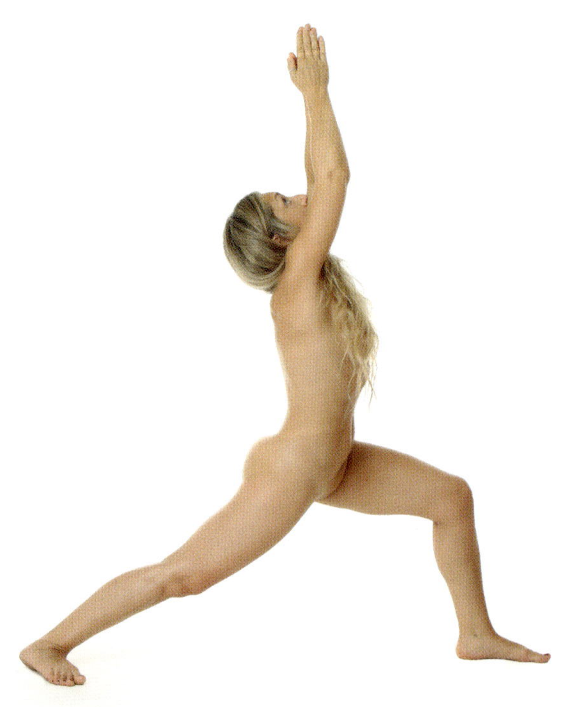

Warrior 1 Pose Left Leg

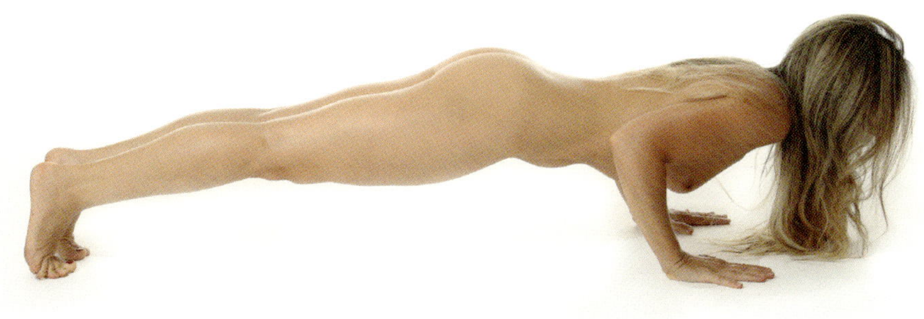

Four-Limbed Staff Pose

13. Four-Limbed Staff Pose

Sanskrit name: *Chaturanga Dandasana* (chaht-tour-ANG-ah don-DAHS-anna)

Meaning: *Chaturanga* = four limbs, *danda* = staff (refers to the spine, the central 'staff' or support of the body), *asana* = posture/pose

Benefits from practising the Four-Limbed Staff Pose regularly:

Builds strength in the arms and wrists

Firms up your abdominal muscles

Skip if: You have carpal tunnel syndrome

How to practise:

Step 1: From Warrior 1 Pose Left Leg *(Virabhadrasana I)*, bring the palms back down to the ground and step back into a plank position.

Step 2: Bring your hands below your shoulders, squeeze your buttocks and activate your abdominal muscles to release tension from your spine, make sure your whole body is in one straight line.

Step 3: Slowly lower your torso and your legs down to the ground, hugging your ribs with your elbows (keep them close to your body throughout).

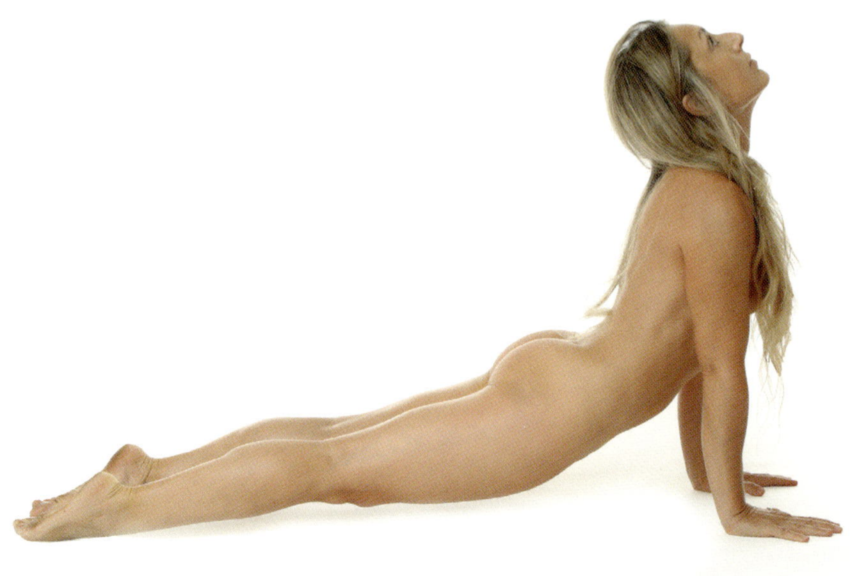

Upward Facing Dog Pose

Step 4: Make sure not to collapse in your shoulders, keep them activated and the space between the shoulder blades broad, look forward.

Tip: If you are a beginner or have not built up enough strength yet, lower your knees down onto the floor.

14. Upward Facing Dog

Sanskrit name: *Urdhva Mukha Shvanasana* (OORD-vah MOO-kah shvon-AHS-anna)

Meaning: *Urdhva* = up/upwards, *mukha* = face, *shvana* = dog, *asana* = posture/pose

Benefits from practising Upward Facing Dog Pose regularly:

Shapes the buttocks, strengthens the spine, arms and wrists

Stretches the front torso and lungs, stimulates the abdominal organs

Aids in relieving fatigue, mild depression and sciatica

Skip if: You have an injured back or carpal tunnel syndrome

How to practise:

Step 1: From Four-Limbed Staff Pose *(Chaturanga Dandasana)*, push the floor away and lean into the palms of your hands.

Step 2: Bring your shoulders back and down, away from your ears and open your chest.

Step 3: Squeeze your buttocks really hard to avoid pressure on your lower back and imagine you are holding a yoga block with your thighs (or actually put one between them and squeeze).

Step 4: Lift the pubis off the ground, only your hands and your legs should be touching it.

Tip: Microbend your elbows to protect your joints.

15. Downward Facing Dog

Sanskrit name: *Adho Mukha Shvanasana* (AH-doh MOO-kah shvah-NAHS-anna)

Meaning: *Adho* = downward, *mukha* = face, *shvana* = dog, *asana* = posture/pose

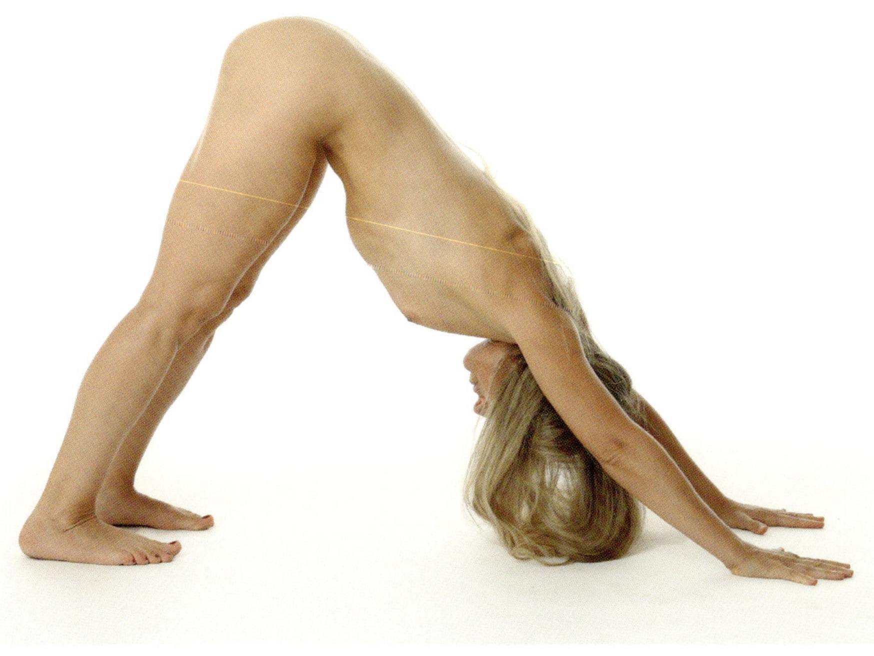

Downward Facing Dog Pose

Benefits from practising Downward Facing Dog regularly:

Relieves headaches, stress, fatigue and mild depression

Stretches shoulders, hamstrings, calves and hands

Strengthens arms and legs

Aids in relieving menopause symptoms as well as menstrual discomfort

Supports a healthy digestion

Beneficial for asthma, sciatica and sinusitis

Skip if: You suffer from carpal tunnel syndrome or diarrhoea

How to practise:

Step 1: From Upward Facing Dog *(Urdhva Mukha Shvanasana)*, press your hands into the ground and lift your torso up towards the ceiling.

Step 2: Push back, lower your heels down on the ground (or near it), keep your legs straight (without locking them); if necessary, bend them slightly.

Step 3: Lift your sitting bones towards the ceiling and activate your abdominal muscles.

Step 4: Push the floor away with your hands and keep your head between your arms (don't let it hang, it should be aligned with your spine).

Tip: Don't get obsessed with getting your feet all the way down to the ground; instead, focus on having a good form.

16. Standing Half-Forward Bend

Sanskrit name: *Ardha Uttanasana* (are-dah oot-tan-AHS-anna)

Meaning: *Ardha* = half, *uttana* = intense stretch/straight, *asana* = posture/pose

Benefits from practising Standing Half-Forward Bend regularly:

Stretches front torso

Improves posture

Strengthens back

Skip if: You have a back injury and be cautious with neck problems

How to practise:

Step 1: From Downward Facing Dog *(Adho Mukha Shvanasana)*, look forward between your hands and step forward onto your mat one foot at a time, you can place the palms of your hands on your shins or keep your arms vertical to the floor.

Step 2: Bring your spine parallel to the floor, your head is an extension of it.

Tip: Microbend your knees to avoid locking them.

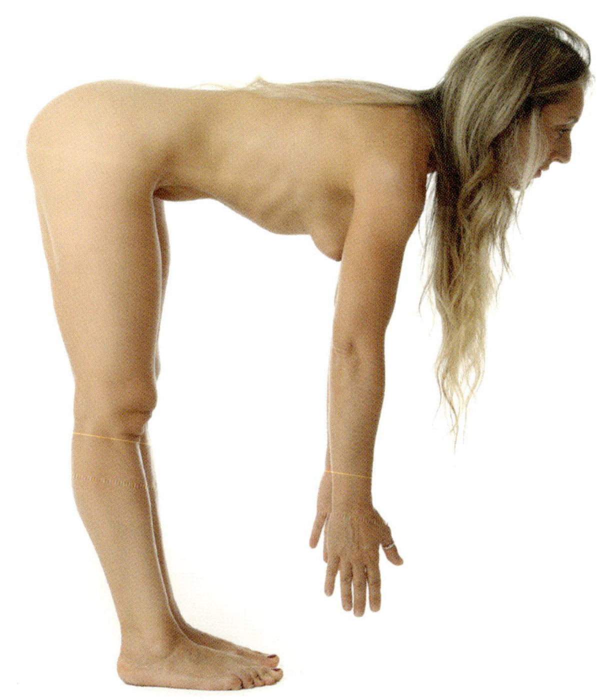

Standing Half-Forward Bend

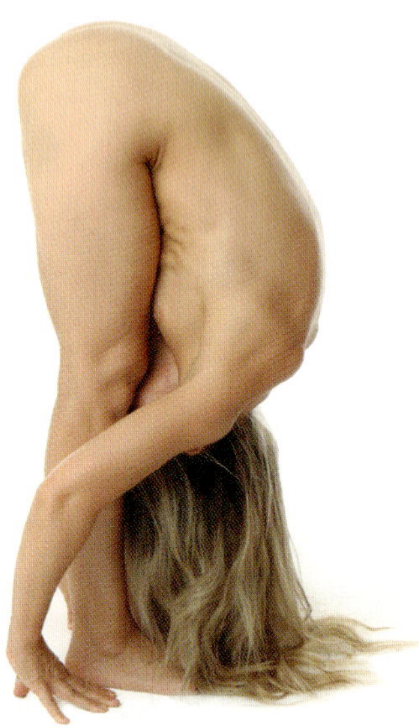

Standing Forward Fold

17. Standing Forward Fold

Sanskrit name: *Uttanasana* (OOT-tan-AHS-ahna)

Meaning: Stretched posture, *uttana* = intense stretch/straight, *asana* = posture/pose

Benefits from practising Standing Forward Fold regularly:

Calms the nervous system and aids in relieving stress, fatigue and mild anxiety

Stimulates the liver and kidneys and supports good digestion

Strengthens thighs, stretches hamstrings, calves and hips

Aids in relieving menopause symptoms

Beneficial for asthma, high blood pressure, headaches and insomnia

Skip if: You have a back injury

How to practise:

Step 1: From Standing Half-Forward Bend *(Ardha Uttanasana)*, relax your back and fold it forwards, let your neck hang.

Step 2: If possible, place the palms of your hands flat on the ground in front of your feet, alternatively let them hang and reach for the ground.

Tip: When folding forward make sure to avoid locking your knees; if necessary, bend your knees ever so slightly.

18. Chair Pose

Sanskrit name: *Utkatasana* (OOT-kah-TAHS-anna)

Meaning: Wild or difficult posture/power posture, *utkata* = wild/intense/powerful/fierce/difficult, *asana* = posture/pose

Benefits of practising Chair Pose regularly:

Strengthens ankles, thighs, calves, feet and spine

Stretches shoulders and chest

Stimulates abdominal organs, diaphragm and heart

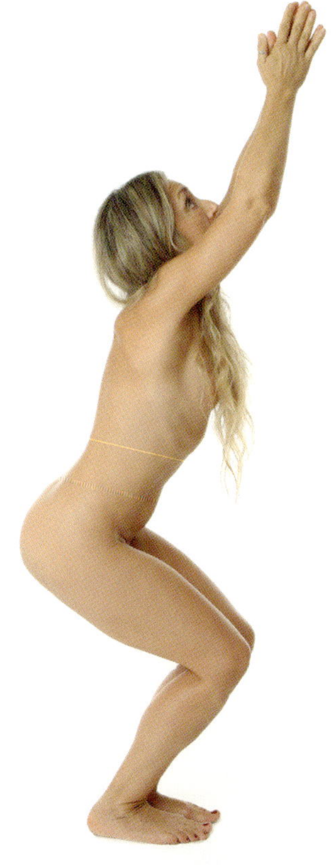

Chair Pose

Skip if: You suffer from insomnia or low blood pressure

How to practise:

Step 1: From Standing Forward Fold *(Uttanasana)*, raise your arms up until they align with your spine, palms facing inwards and bend your knees.

Step 2: Lower your buttocks down slowly, activate your core.

Step 3: Keep the lower back long by taking your tailbone down towards the ground and in towards your pubis.

Tip: Squeeze your knees together for extra support in this posture.

19. Mountain Pose

Sanskrit name: *Tadasana* (tah-DAHS-anna)

Meaning: *Tada* = mountain, *asana* = posture/pose

Deepen your breath and focus on your feet. Feel the connection to the ground beneath and pay attention to your weight distribution. Do you have more weight on one foot or in a certain part of your feet? Scan your whole body and feel the sensations that arise.

Benefits from practising Mountain Pose regularly:

Strengthens thighs, knees and feet

Helps to improve posture

Firms up the abdomen and buttocks

Relieves sciatica

Skip if: You suffer from insomnia or low blood pressure

How to practise:

Step 1: From Chair Pose *(Utkatasana),* lower your arms and straighten your body. Stand with your feet parallel to each other, big toes slightly touching.

Step 2: Lift your toes, spread them and lower them back down to the ground, rock sideways and back and forth, distribute your weight evenly and come to a standstill.

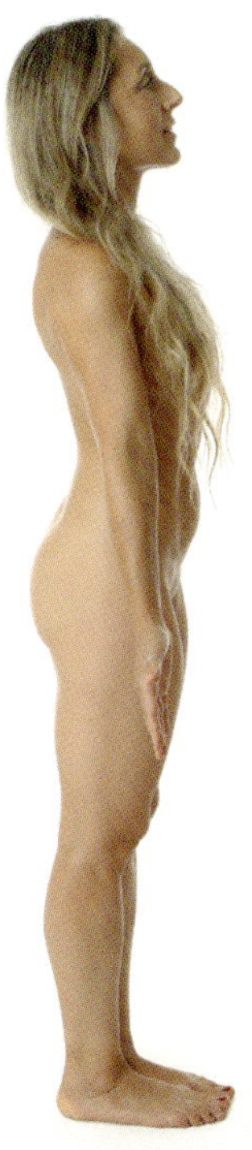

Mountain Pose

Step 3: Bring your pelvis into a neutral position by picturing a bucket of water and finding the perfect position where the water doesn't overflow.

Step 4: Bring your head back a bit and make a slight double-chin to align it with your spine, then let your arms hang beside your body.

Tip: At the end of your Sun Salutation *(Surya Namaskar)* B practice, spend at least 5 minutes lying on the ground on your back in Corpse Pose *(Shavasana)* to enjoy and benefit from deep relaxation.

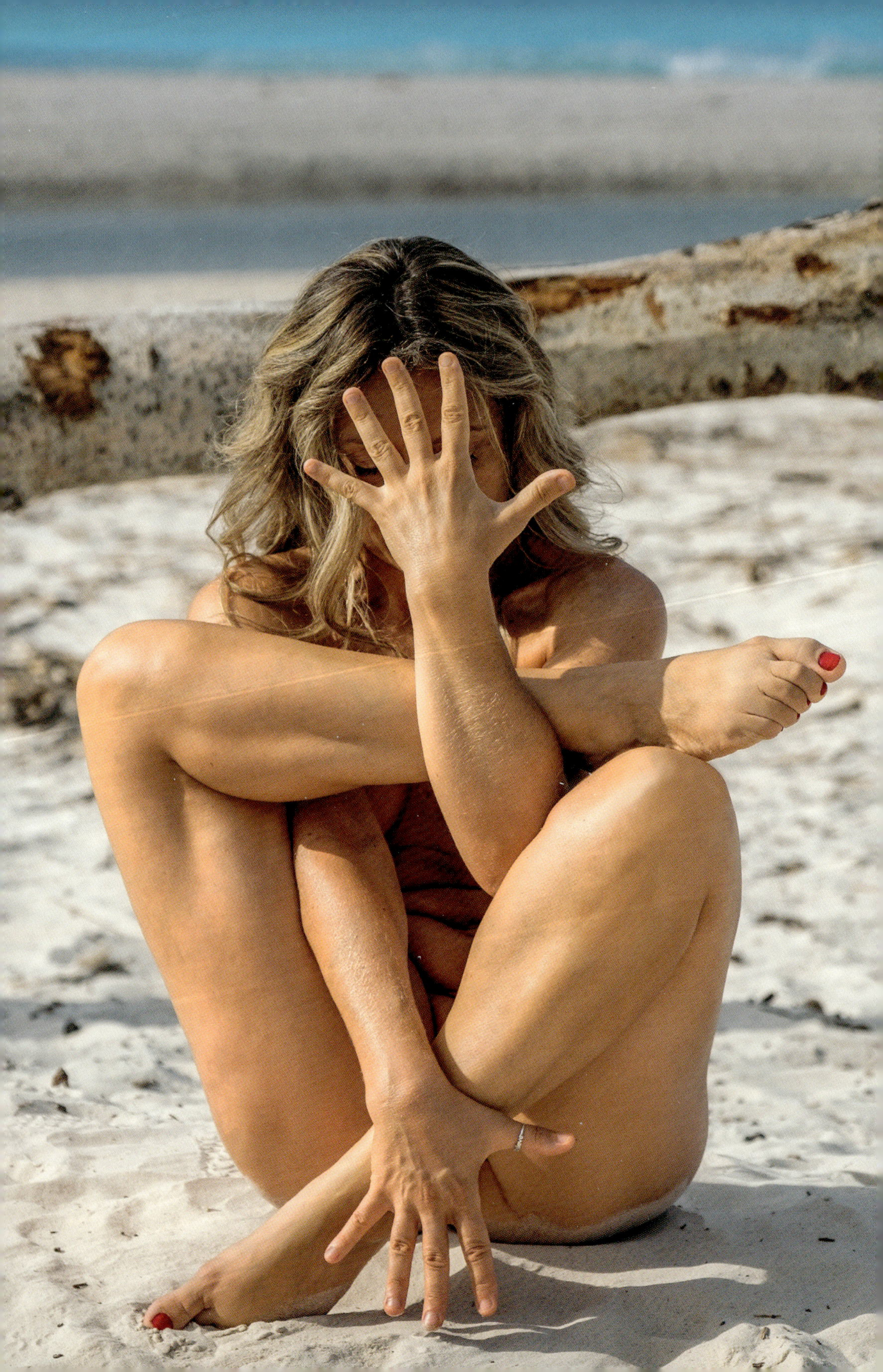

PART FOUR

What They Say

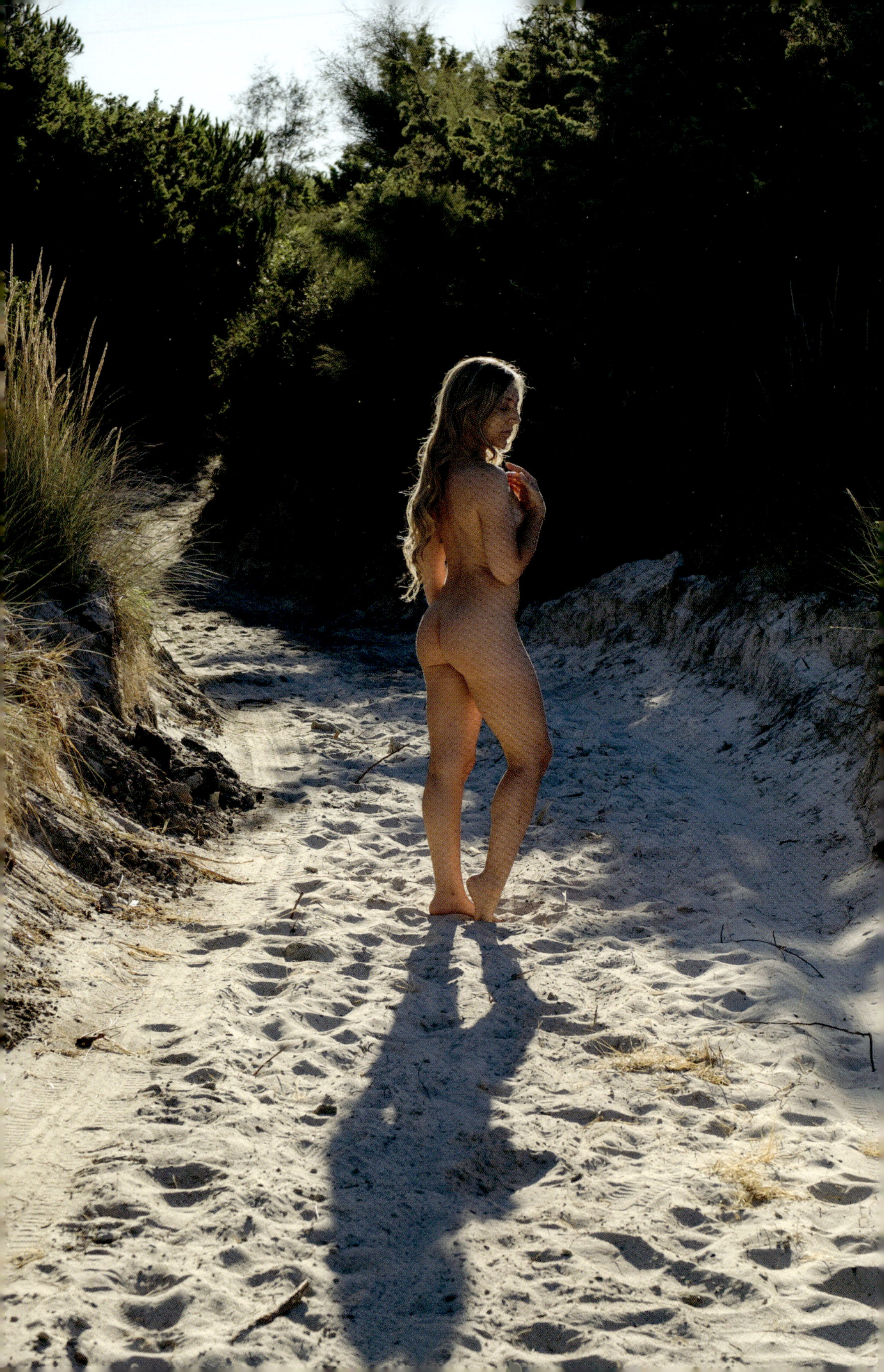

CHAPTER 17

Student Feedback

In this chapter I include feedback from some of my students whom I affectionately refer to as my 'Doritos'. By sharing their experiences of taking naked yoga classes, I hope to allay any concerns or worries you might have about attending a class.

Stella D

What was your situation before starting the class?

I knew I was overweight and lethargic and had been looking for a new activity to help me regain my fitness. I had been on many naturist holidays and had once, many years ago, enjoyed yoga so was intrigued at combining the two.

What have been the results?

Doria's classes are an excellent workout. She gives you different options for different levels of expertise. I love the way she manages to make it challenging without it being competitive. After a few weeks of practising I could feel my body becoming stronger, firmer and more supple. In addition, my energy levels began to increase.

Gary O

What was your situation before starting the class?

My health and general wellbeing were poor – very out of shape and suffering with joint and back pain. My stomach had issues due to my sedentary lifestyle at the time. Mentally, I was feeling a bit depressed, isolated, and was looking for a class-based activity that fits into my naturist values, to be more social, and address the health problems that were creeping up on me.

What have been the results?

My stomach feels so much better after the classes, working on core muscles as well as the dynamic flows has helped me more than previous medication. I don't feel as bloated or getting tight stomach cramps anymore. Maybe it helps to de-stress me which also adds to positive benefits on my stomach area. I feel like it's completely changed my outlook on what yoga can do for the mind and body.

Hazel B

What was your situation before starting the class?

My situation before I started naked yoga was that I had recently left an 18-year marriage in which we shared very little intimacy. Before leaving I had already started a process of overhauling my life as my health and wellbeing were disastrously low. Having overhauled my life and made many changes I moved to London and embarked on a journey of trying to undo as many of the suppressive messages that had led me into an unhappy life as I could. I had already been practising yoga (clothes on) and this had helped me to manage my symptoms of chronic fatigue and joint/muscle pains, etc.

What have been the results?

Feeling more at ease with my body, feeling like everyone else will like my body if they've got any sense, wearing the clothes I've always wanted to and loving and appreciating my body! Achieving a headstand was very momentous for me. It really gave me a sense of body confidence to feel that my body could manage this. I feel strong and proud that I have accomplished this skill.

Francesca S

What was your situation before starting the class?

When you spend half of your teenage years counting calories and obsessively checking the scales, the way you look at yourself and at your body is all but normal. Eating disorders, and in my own case, anorexia, kept hitting me back in the difficult moments of my life, when controlling food and weight was the only form of control I had on events. I was never too skinny, but in reality, what I felt was 'not good enough, smart enough, accepted enough'.

I 'bumped' into Doria and her naked yoga practice after years of all-consuming and mostly unsuccessful psychotherapy. If you reject your body, the very last thing you want to do is stand in front of a group of people exposing every centimetre of your naked shield. But I knew Doria's story and, the first time I met her, I could not help myself from searching in her abdomen for the pale, thin scar she was effortlessly showing. We all have scars: some very visible, others hidden to the sight of many.

She was so natural and relaxed, so reassuring and strong that I followed her movements as if hypnotised. It didn't take long before feeling a renewed energy filling my body: I could *see* my hands, my legs, my tummy, everything of me as the real myself. After years of unacceptance, I slowly started looking at my body without separating my 'inside' from my 'outside'. I was finally moving in the world with and through my body, perceiving it no longer as other than me.

What have been the results?

Doria taught me to be kind to myself, to accept the person I became and to love that person. Life is such an incredible journey and I feel privileged to walk with bare feet into life with such an incredible teacher.

Michael W

What was your situation before starting the class?

I first entered Doria's naked yoga class four years ago. I was at a low point in my life, depression, the demise of my marriage and my searching for the elusive, as time runs short…

Despite Doria's 'body positive' campaigning, it wasn't particularly relevant for me. I was already a long-time nudist and life model and was always comfortable (if not more so) naked than clothed. But my yoga practice was a spiritual and meditative experience for me, and my life modelling was likewise, so naked yoga seemed like a natural combination.

So from my very first class, I placed my mat directly opposite Doria. That was *my* spot: I want to learn and receive the energy transfer from the most spiritual person in the room, and so from that day forward we always practise facing each other and in Warrior 2 Pose with our arms and fingers, strong and outstretched, I feel her uplifting energy 'jump' across the room and enter my body through my fingertips, and energise *me*, physically and emotionally. For me our connection is palpable when on our mats.

Long may we practise together, long may we be a part of each other's lives, long may we be 'partners in crime', celebrating the beauty and naturalness of the naked human body.

Betty

What was your situation before starting the class?

Most of my life had passed me by, being occupied by work and career that I wasn't passionate about. About ten years ago, I left a corporate job to start my own business. I married my husband six years ago. We travelled extensively. As an 'older couple', soon after we married, we decided to start IVF. Life had not prepared me for the ups and downs and emotional roller-coaster ride of IVF. After many attempts and a miscarriage, we had to face the fact that we were not going to have children.

My life had stagnated. I felt like I was not doing anything meaningful with my life. I felt like I had failed as a woman. Nothing could pull me away from the rut I was in. Then in July 2020, I was diagnosed with DCIS (pre-cancer or stage 0) in both breasts. This was a big reality check for me. Life was telling me I was not immortal.

Melbourne was in the middle of a strict lockdown due to Covid-19. I knew I wanted to get healthy and build up my sense of self to prepare me for what was to come. I searched locally for yoga classes, but I could not find anyone in Australia that I could connect with. I had just about given up when my husband found Doria Yoga. I was rapt to see Doria offered naked yoga sessions via zoom. Online classes were the perfect set up for me.

Doria's website mentioned her story and that she had undergone cancer. I was inspired. Doria looked amazing. My goal was to calm my mind, build confidence and start to have a more body positive image of myself. Plus, I needed to improve my flexibility. Instantly, I was at ease in Doria's class. Each time I have logged into the class, Doria is there as a shining light.

I had breast-conserving surgery in October 2020. I had missed a few yoga classes, and I couldn't wait to get back into my yoga practice. I feel classes are somehow deeper and more liberating by being naked. My scars are visible, but I don't mind. I have embraced them.

What have been the results?

It has helped me to be inspired and stay more positive about life. I am less conscious about my body and I do not scrutinize it as much. I am accepting myself, flaws and all.

How was it practising yoga online compared to in person?

I much prefer practicing yoga online. It doesn't feel so in your face. I feel there is a respect between the people and less focus on the physical body.

Did you like working with people from around the world?

It is wonderful that people join from around the world. Everyone is so friendly and focused on practising their yoga. We are a bunch of diverse people, but at the end of the day, we are all still part of the same human race.

Laurie

What was your situation before starting the class?

My life has been very turbulent from my teenage years, I struggled with my mental health. In the darkest depths of depression I couldn't see the light. I was unable to see colour in the world and some days getting out of bed was the hardest task imaginable. I was so weak and felt so alone, trapped inside my darkness. At one stage, I didn't want to be here anymore and I battled with difficult intrusive thoughts. The beauty of nature was invisible, the sun was no longer warm, the taste of food was bland, rest was no longer rest and greeting cards would cause me to break down in tears as it was too overwhelming.

I grew up with a lot of pressure on body image and weight. I was in a competitive industry where good was never good enough and the scales were often the first thing you stepped on. I was fortunate to have never suffered an eating disorder but weight did cause me anxiety and I never felt good enough in my own skin for who I was.

I was raped ten years ago which has been an ongoing healing process. For many years I put so much blame on myself and pushed away the reality of what had happened. I couldn't even name it or say the word "rape" aloud. I have cried so many tears, had the scariest of flashbacks and undertaken EMDR (Eye Movement Desensitization and Reprocessing) therapy as part of my healing process. Coming to terms with the fact that it wasn't my fault and it shouldn't have happened has taken a long time. I remember the evening like yesterday if I really think back but I wonder if they even recall my name or who I was.

I was working through a lot of personal trauma at the time of starting yoga with Doria and had some previous experience of yoga.

What has the process been like?

I have really enjoyed the classes I have taken to date and I have felt very calm and in tune with my body. It's helped me to accept my flaws and who I am as a person. I recall in my first naked yoga class looking at a roll of skin and then breathing into this and thinking this is who I am. I became more and more appreciative of my body and what it could achieve rather than worrying about any area that I may not have liked on myself as much. It has also been a very safe place to be naked with other women and men. It has made me question the vulnerability of humans. How as a society we have put such a heavy weighting on clothing and identity when we were all born naked.

What have been the results?

Taking time out to be mindful and work with my body. The body holds the score and learning to be more in tune with what my body is telling me has definitely developed through yoga. I have also felt challenged in the classes which I have liked. This challenge has always been the right amount.

How has practising online helped you during lockdown?

I took some classes during lockdown and this helped me to fit some self-care into working from home. I enjoyed being in a zen zone away from the worries of Covid for the class.

How was it practising yoga online compared to in person?

I preferred in person for the sense of community and seeing others in person. However I think being online enables me to focus just as much if not more on my own body and movement. It was great to not have any travelling to and from class. Furthermore, it was nice to have my own candles burning and home comforts when practising at home.

Did you like working with people from around the world?

Yes I did; it was lovely to feel part of the wider community. We were all going through the same thing but experiencing this in a different way.

Doria also takes the time at the end of the class for any questions and I know that she would be there between classes if I had a concern.

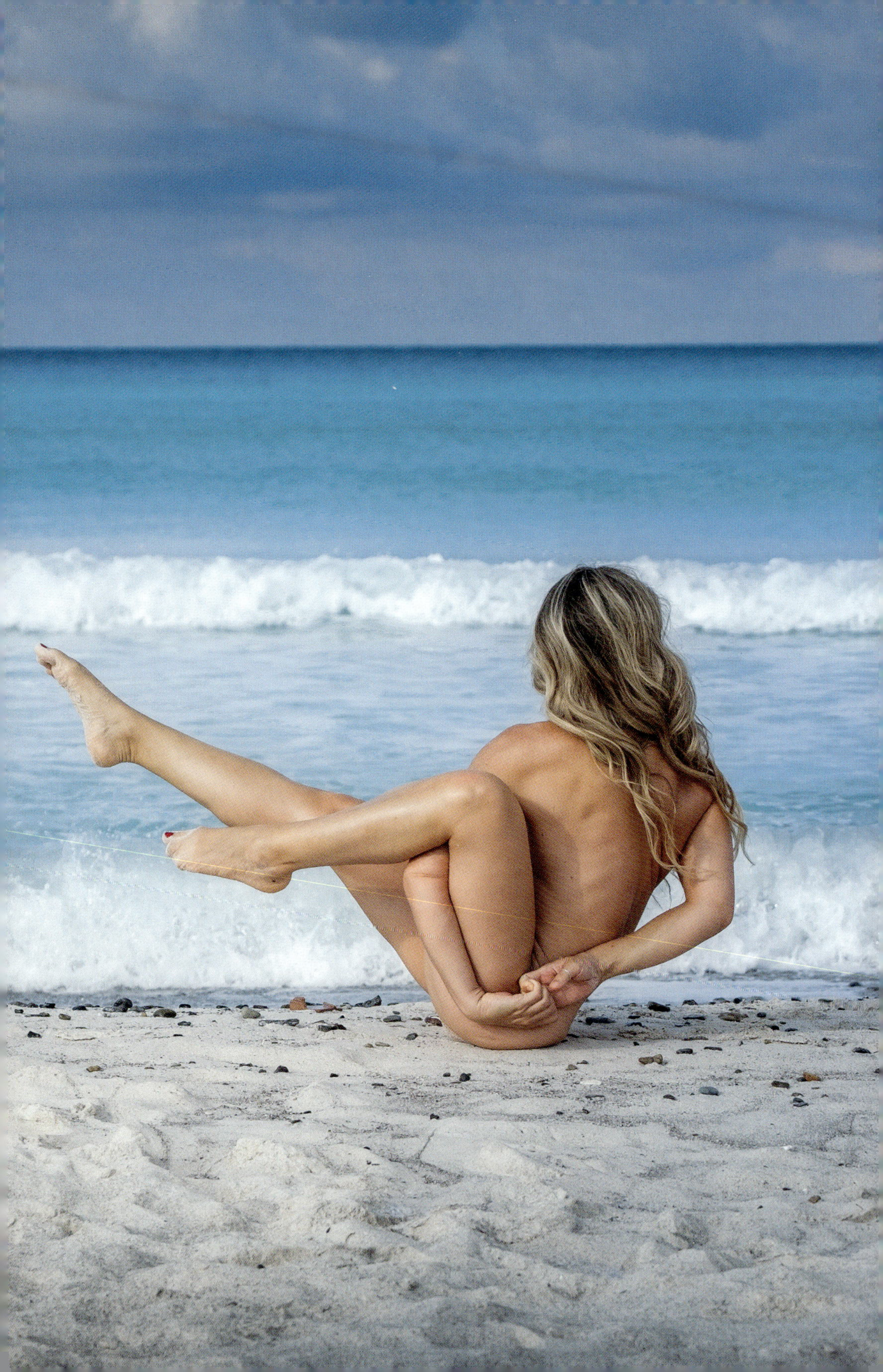

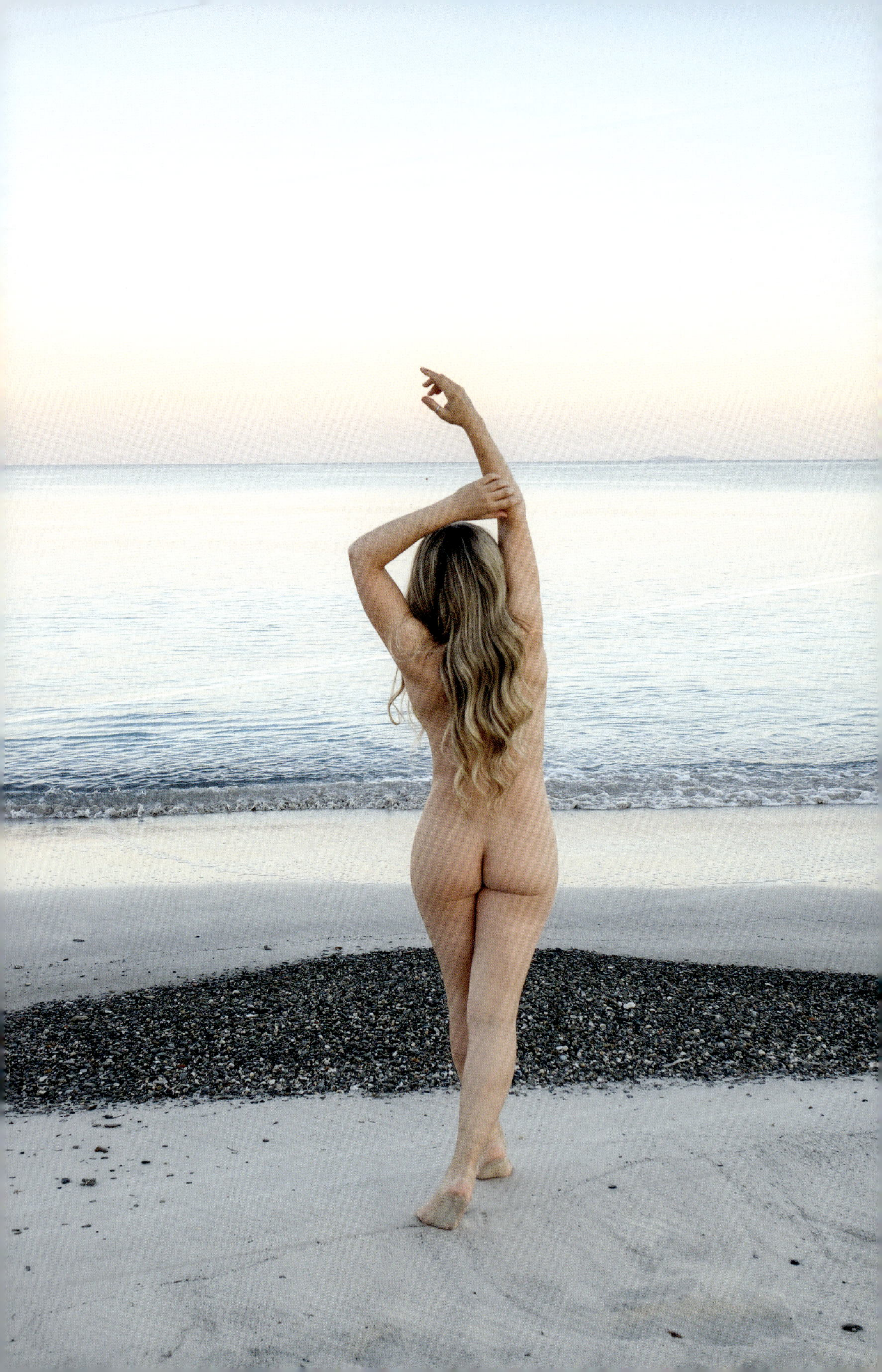

CHAPTER 18

Endnote

"Naturally, obviously, nudity is a part of life."
– Theo James

I hope that you have enjoyed reading my journey and that you may have benefited from following the Beginners' Yoga Guide. I hope that you will feel inspired also to get naked and stay naked, even if only in the privacy of your own home or garden.

What I have learned from my battle with cancer and life in general is that we need to embrace all that has happened in our history, both the good and the bad. These experiences have formed us into the person we are today. To love ourselves fully we need to accept our past mishaps and mistakes and be thankful to those who have helped us or raised us up. Equally, we need to understand and forgive those who have hurt us, or put obstacles in our way.

The past will never be resolved by any amount of hatred, remorse or regret. By learning to truly love our bodies – bumps, warts, injuries, deformities and all – we can let go of our mental suffering and open ourselves to giving and receiving love.

If you'd like to know more about getting naked then you can join the Naturist Society to read about the history and philosophy behind nudism. They have many resources on their website including a magazine and a list of beaches where you can go nude in the US: www.naturistsociety.com. There is also the British Naturist Society at www.bn.org.uk and other naturist groups and organizations around the world. If you're now ready to join a Naked Yoga Class, there are groups in most cities.

I offer one-to-one sessions, group classes and individual coaching online. You can follow me on social media or find out more on my website: www.doriayoga.com.

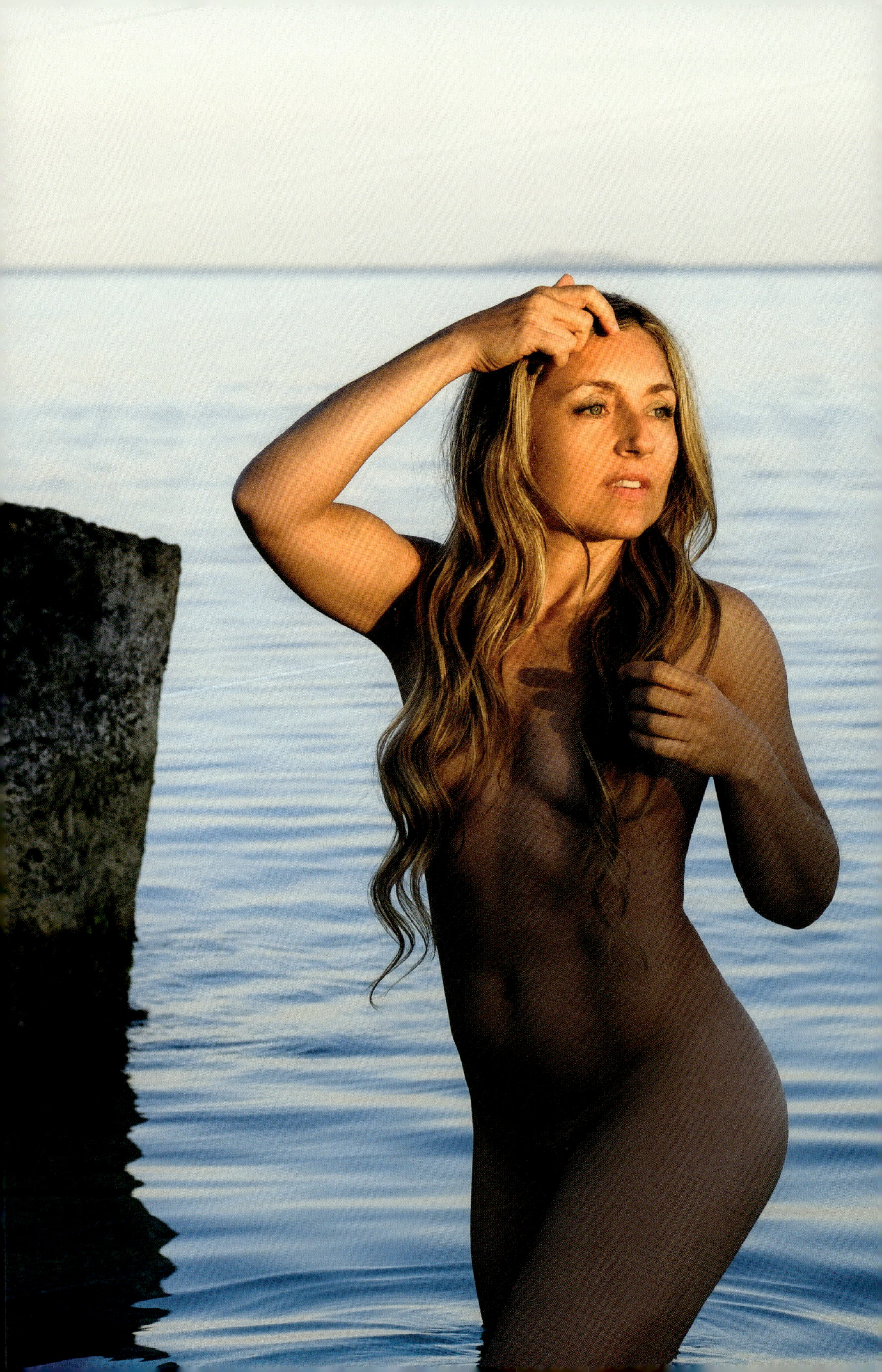

INDEX

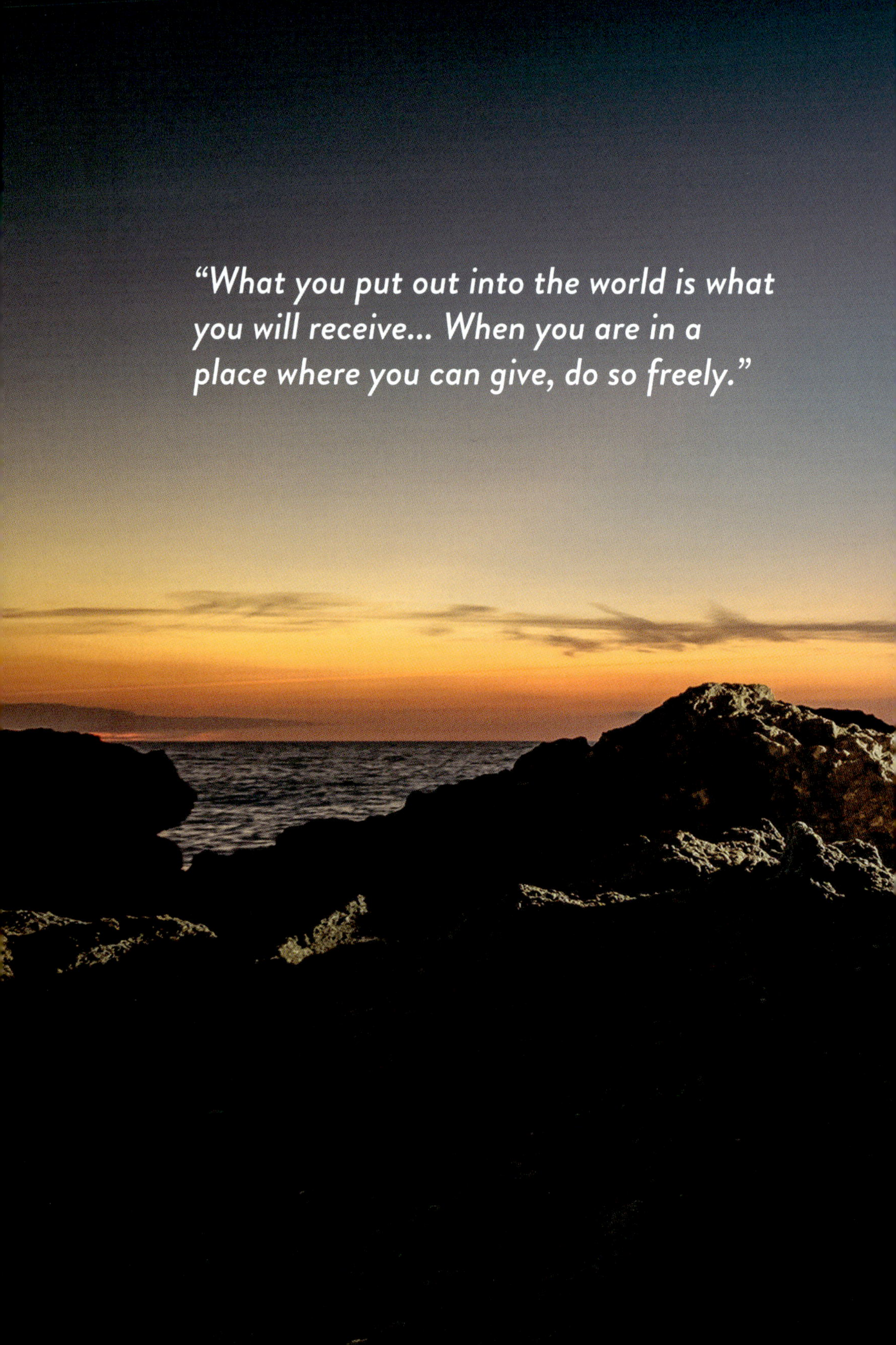

"What you put out into the world is what you will receive... When you are in a place where you can give, do so freely."

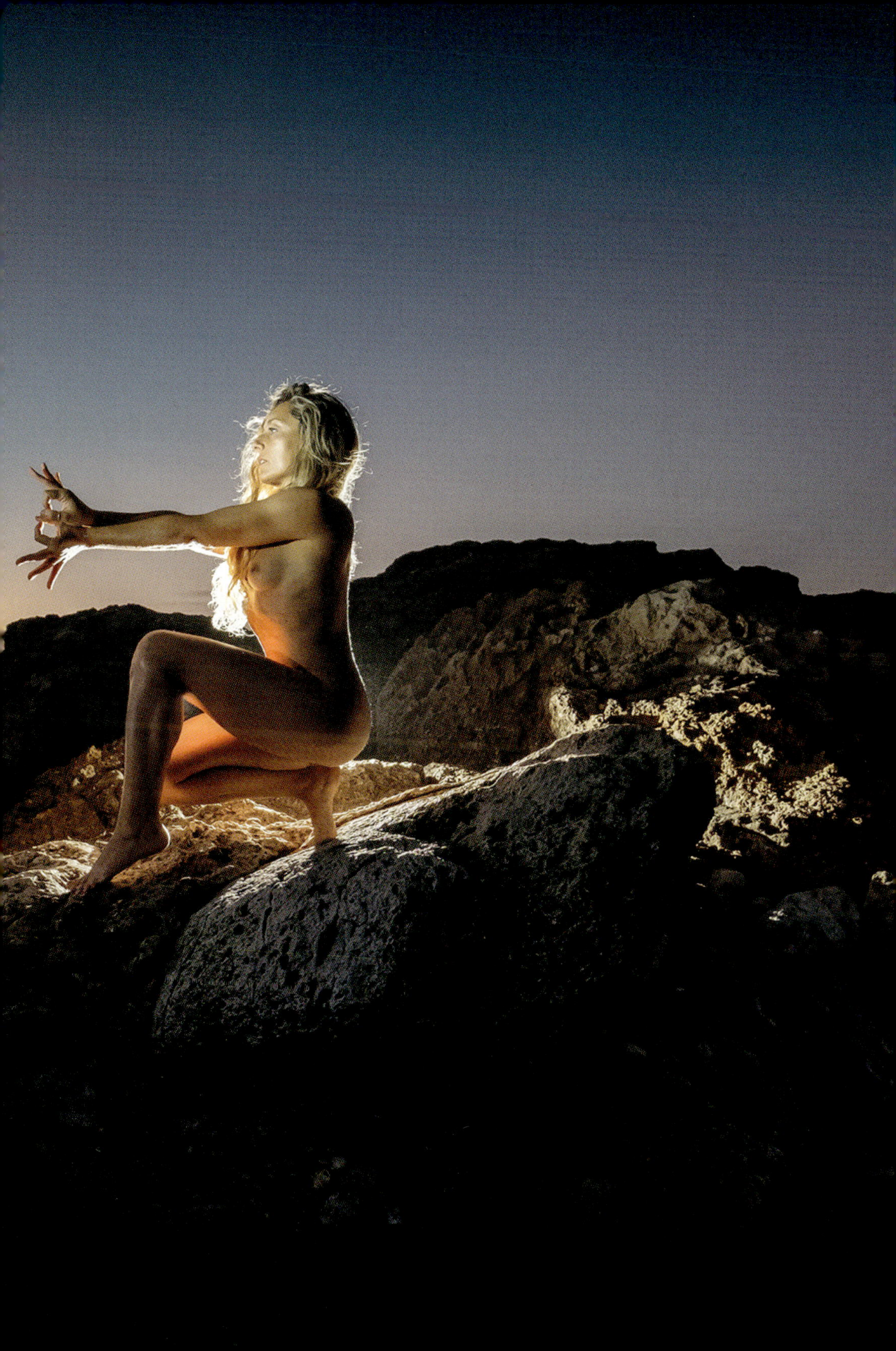

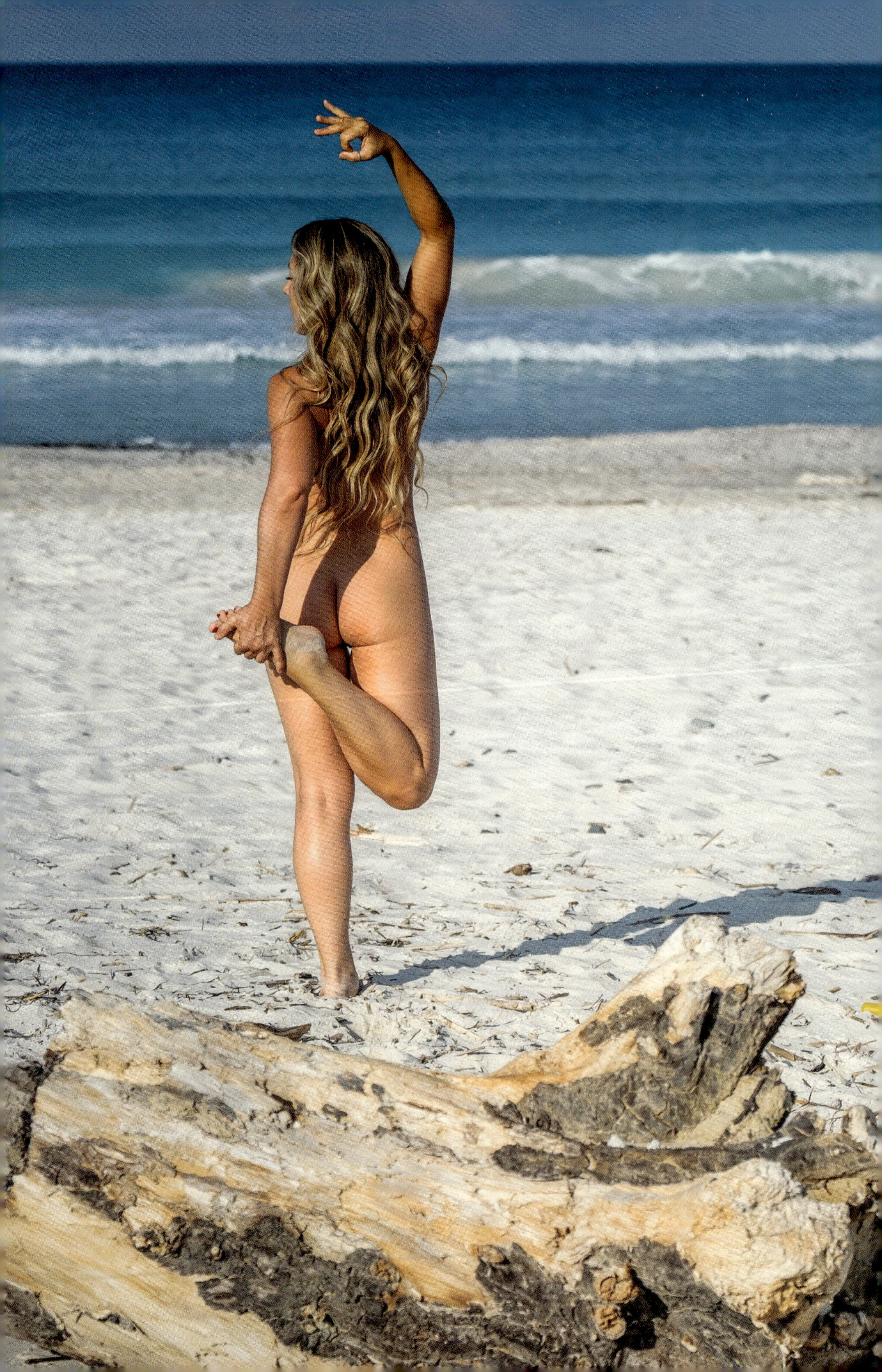